THE WAY BACK

THE WAY BACK

HEAL YOUR SELF • HEAL THE WORLD

SAM ROSE, C.N. M.S.

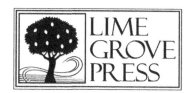

LIME
GROVE
PRESS

The Way Back
Heal Your Self • Heal The World

Cover art and design
Paul Manchester/FugitiveColors.com

ISBN: 0615516033
ISBN-13: 9780615516035
LCCN: 2011935007
Lime Grove Press, Los Angeles, California

for Merry and Zoë

FOREWORD

Last month, we scattered Nate's ashes in Carmel Valley, in a secluded field of wild rye grass and spring flowers. As our impromptu ceremony got under way, a breeze came up off the Pacific to sweep away the lingering fog, and our small group warmed in the midday sun.

We were young, old, rich, poor, influential and regular folk, most of us Nate's former students, drawn by our love for the man and our gratitude for his generosity. Zoë took the red-eye from NYU and flew up with Merry and me. Heather drove down from UC Davis where she's a professor of agronomy now. Al cancelled one of his popular slide shows to be there.

Following Nate's last wishes, the three dozen of us each took a handful of his ashes out into the field and spread them in a place we felt especially drawn to. I ended up nearly a quarter of a mile from our circle, at a bent oak that stood where the valley nestled against the mountains.

When we returned, we found that Noah had somehow prepared a picnic feast for us all. No one could figure out how he pulled it off. He arrived with no supplies, we were miles from the nearest town, and he didn't drive—Maggie had given him a lift from Santa Monica. But those of us who knew him were used to this sort of little miracle.

We spent the afternoon talking about our lessons with Nate and how they had changed the direction of our personal and professional lives. I heard many stories that day that left me with a renewed sense of hope.

But the full effect of his passing didn't register until I was on the plane heading home, gazing at the fragile landscape twenty thousand feet below.

Nate was really gone.

He would never again take a lost person under his wing and teach him how to live an authentic and vibrant life, never lead another misguided soul back to the truth about his powerful connection to this planet, or open our eyes to the perilous course we humans have set for ourselves.

To reach the critical mass necessary to alter that course, more people would have to hear his message and let it change them. With Nate silent now and so much still to be done, I couldn't ignore that little voice in my head anymore—the one that for nearly two decades had been telling me the day would come when I'd have to stop playing it small, disseminating bits and pieces of Nate's wisdom in the relative safety of my nutrition office.

It was time to step out of my fiercely guarded comfort zone and go public.

It was time to tell my story.

THE WAY BACK

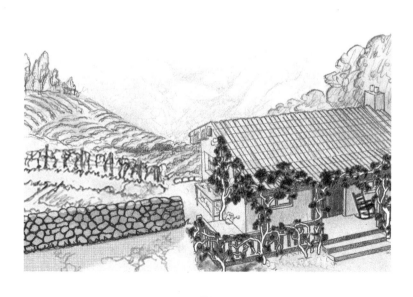

ONE

I groped for the bottle of Pepto Bismol on the nightstand, and a sharp pain shot under my shoulder blades. I collapsed back onto the bed, exhausted.

You could sum up the "wild revelry" of the night before in one word: colic. That's what the doctor called it. Our four-month-old, Zoë, was up at all hours, and for Merry and me, sleep had become elusive and precious. One of our more colorful friends insisted that the baby's distress was the result of unopened chakras. Whatever it was, we were up with her a half dozen times.

By all rights, I should've been unconscious for another three or four hours, but I couldn't unwind. I owed songs to five or six producers, and I'd been in a spin for weeks. All I could coax out of my guitar these days were old folk and blues tunes from college—a far cry from anything resembling a pop song.

To make it in the music business, you have to keep paddling out to the waves with the faith that you'll eventually catch a big one. I'd always been that guy, confident and optimistic, buoyed up by near misses and the occasional tune that caught on. I never thought much about the other 90 percent of it, the failures, the long, long dry spells, the dozens of songs my twin brother Geoffrey and I had written and pitched that would never see the light of day. I'd always been good at the necessary delusion. But a baby wailing in the next room is all about reality. She needed everything… food and insurance, strollers and toys. Private school, maybe. Piano lessons. College. How in the hell would we manage that? Living in L.A. on a musician's erratic income was hard enough *without* a child!

There was low-level panic quietly shrieking through me all the time.

Evidently, desperation and creativity don't mix well. Over the last few months, the reliable stream of music that played in my mind for decades had been slowing to a trickle. Now it was completely dry. Sure, mediocre, even good ideas would come. But when you're trying to sell songs at the top of the music business, good isn't good enough. Great is all that matters. And you can't force great. Great drops into your head out of the ether—a killer melody or instrumental hook that sets a song apart and makes people listen.

Nothing close to great had "dropped" in months, not a single idea worth putting on tape, and it was torture going back into my home studio for another day of staring at Geoffrey's lyrics and willing them to sing to me.

The irony was we were doing all right. We finally had a hit on the charts. Doors were opening for us, and even so, I couldn't make myself believe that it would last. In the middle of the night, the weight on my chest was crushing.

❧

I struggled out of bed and headed for the shower. I took care stepping into the tub—having recently wrenched my back with that simple act—and let the hot spray unkink a few knots.

The water streamed off the high curve of my belly. *A beer gut? When did that happen?*

I couldn't remember the last time I'd felt healthy.

When the water went cold, I shut it off and whispered a small, desperate prayer—or the unpracticed amateur equivalent: "If anyone's listening, I could really use some help. I need a spark. I'm just not feeling it anymore. What the hell am I supposed to do?"

A final droplet plunged into the draining tub. Its soft *ping* reverberated in the shower's hollow acoustics.

❧

After squeezing into a pair of jeans, I put on a pot of coffee and opened the morning paper, turning the pages almost hypnotically. The print blurred for a second, and when I blinked to refocus, a curious little ad in the lower right corner of a page caught my attention.

When you're ready
Call: 310-555-8835

3

Ready for what?

I turned the page.

There it was again. This time the ad was perched in the upper right corner. Two more of the little blurbs sat parked at the bottom of the facing page, just left and right of center. It was a transparent ploy, this fake mystery, probably to get people to buy something. On page twenty, there were four of them, arranged at the edges like the points of a compass. "When you're ready, call. When you're ready, call. When you're ready, call. When you're ready..."

As I scanned the rest of the paper, there were more and more of the little ads—seemingly hundreds of them glaring up at me.

I squeezed my eyes shut, took a few deep breaths, and looked again.

The newspaper lay open to page 16, where I'd seen the first ad. There it sat, in its corner spot. But when I rifled through the paper in search of the clones, they were gone.

What the hell? I *really* needed some sleep.

I turned back to page 16 and stared at the ad's top line.

When you're ready

Obviously, I was ready for something. My body, my whole life needed something, and I had no clue what it might be. But as I sat looking at the ad, a distinct and rare sense of clarity came over me. A sense of surrender.

I poured myself a cup of coffee, picked up the phone, and dialed the number.

TWO

"Yes, hello." The man on the other end was all business. I introduced myself. "I saw your ad in the paper and—"

"So, you're ready then," he cut me off.

I moved my finger to the phone's cradle and considered hanging up. Instead, I asked, "So, who are you?"

"The name's Nathan. Call me Nate."

"And what exactly do you do, Nate? Are you some sort of psychologist?"

"The label's not important. What I do is show the truth to folks who are ready to make the most of their lives." He waited a moment, and then added, "Are you making the most of yours?"

"Well, not exactly."

"Then maybe we should get together."

I paused as alarms went off in my head. *Who IS this nutcase? What if he's a con man, or worse?* But over all the what-ifs, a less familiar internal voice chimed in: *You need all the help you can get. Take it!*

I grabbed a pen and notebook from the kitchen counter.

"Okay," I said. "I'd like to make an appointment."

"No appointment necessary. Feel free to stop by whenever the sun's up."

"And your fee, what do you charge?"

"We can talk about compensation later."

Ah—the catch. But I kept writing as Nate gave me directions to his house above Topanga Canyon. He said he looked forward to our meeting and hung up before I could say another word.

I settled at the kitchen table over a second cup of coffee, and soon my mind took a familiar turn, wandering back to Zoë and the day she was born.

∽

Merry was already eight days past her due date, so we knew we were taking our chances going all the way to the mall to buy a camera. When her water broke, as if on cue, while we stood at the head of the checkout line, we shouldn't have been surprised—after all, we *were* in Hollywood.

The sun was dropping below the horizon when we arrived at the hospital. It rose and set and rose again before Zoë came, and in all that time, neither of us slept. But we rested together in the room after she arrived, lying on the bed until the doctor stopped in to tell us that the baby's tests were fine and we were free to go.

Merry and I sat in silent elation for a few minutes longer, staring at our beautiful daughter. Then we gathered our things and a nurse pushed Merry and Zoë toward the elevator in a wheelchair.

Walking down the long, sterile corridor, I thought about my own father. I could hardly remember him; he left our family when I was two. Still, he taught me something I'd never forgotten: Only a fool isn't wary. Love will screw with you. I didn't dwell on it, but I could feel myself backing away whenever someone got too close. Now, though, *I* was somebody's father and my love for Zoë poured over that old wound, soothing it.

"I'll get the car," I said and stepped through the opening double doors. As I crossed the parking lot, the midday sun seemed to find every reflective surface. Everything crystallized, and I felt the full weight of what I owed this little girl.

My head throbbed. I couldn't begin to imagine what Merry was going through. Finally, I arrived at our 1984 Volvo sedan and slowly drove back to the hospital's main entrance. We strapped Zoë in and collapsed into the bucket seats. "How about some tunes?" I asked, switching on the radio.

A saxophone wailed over the first few bars of a familiar-sounding track. We looked at each other in disbelief. The song playing was "Nothing but the Radio On," a tune Geoffrey and I co-wrote. Dave Koz recorded the song nearly a year before for Capitol Records, but the label delayed the album so many times, I'd pretty much given up hope for it. I had no idea the record was out—or that our song had been chosen as a single... until now.

"What are the odds..."

"Shhh, let's listen." Merry put one hand on my knee and nudged up the volume.

With our daughter asleep in the backseat, we sat in the circular drive and let the music, my music, wash over us.

෧ඌ

Over a third cup of coffee I tried to persuade myself that I still had a song like that in me. But the passion that kept me going for decades was gone. So was my inner muse. Maybe they'd run off together.

At breakfast, Merry asked if there was any news about our hit.

"Geoffrey says we're still in the Top 20 on *Billboard*. Capitol did an international release a couple of weeks ago and we're number one in Hong Kong."

"Hong Kong?" Merry's voice rose in excitement, punctuating each word. "Number—One—In—Hong—Kong!"

"Yeah," I said.

"God, honey. You're not excited?"

"No, it's good. I'm glad we'll have decent money coming in for a while."

"But what?"

"We've got a few meetings coming up with A&R people who want us to write something for artists they've got in the studio."

"That's terrific!"

"Well, potentially terrific. It's just… I've been sitting on a bunch of Geoffrey's lyrics, and I've got nada. Nothing."

Merry's face softened. "Oh, honey, you've gone through dry spells before. Be patient. It'll be fine, you'll see."

Well, there's dry, and then there's the Sahara.

"The thing is I can't wait around for inspiration anymore. So I'm meeting with a guy today who might be able to help me," I said, without going into how I'd found him.

There was a long, uncomfortable silence.

"Sam…" Merry scanned the ceiling as if the right thing to say was hiding somewhere up there. "I know you've been under a lot of pressure, with the baby and all. If it would help, I could go back to work sooner than we planned."

"No, no, I've got this," I assured her. "Everything is under control."

∾

On my way out of the house, I stopped by the bedroom where Merry sat in our rocking chair nursing the baby. She gave me an anxious look.

"Later on, how about we take Zoë for a walk on the Promenade?" I suggested.

"Sure, it'll be good to get out of the house."

I stroked Zoë's little head. *Her life's so simple. Must be nice.*

I wrapped my arms around my wife and daughter, and the three of us rocked gently for a moment. Then I kissed my girls and headed off to meet Nate.

THREE

It's a short ride up Pacific Coast Highway from Santa Monica to Topanga Canyon. But that morning the marine layer was especially thick, and cars on the road were reduced to ghostly pairs of headlights and taillights. Traffic was moving at a snail's pace.

Finally, I turned off PCH and cautiously zigzagged up the canyon. The dense haze near the top made staying on the road an unnerving challenge. The street narrowed and then stopped in front of a wooded area. I reversed and rolled back to check the address of the last house, but it was a couple of numbers shy of the one Nate had given me.

I craned forward over the steering wheel and stared up at the street's dead end.

Shit. What am I doing here? I should turn around and go home.

But I didn't.

Outside of the car's warm interior, the cool, thick air swirled around the back of my neck. I walked to the end of the street and found the elusive house number, painted on the curb, barely visible under a pile of leaves.

The fog hung thick around the brush, erasing everything more than a few yards away. Pushing aside some low-lying branches, I took a few steps and found myself at the head of a dirt path that led up the mountain to a simple white gate supported by two wooden posts.

Beyond the gate, the path was gravel, and the crunch of shifting rocks amplified my footsteps into the surrounding stillness. I was about to give in to the jitters and turn around when a small, single-story structure materialized at the crest of the hill.

Dark, weathered timber supported the overhanging tile roof and framed the front door of a small Spanish-style home that reminded me of buildings I had seen inside the old missions at Santa Barbara and Carmel.

Two thick jade plants stood guard on either side of the steps leading up to a wide porch. A nursery's worth of clay pots overflowing with greenery splashed yellow, purple, and orange blossoms over the porch railing. Flowering jasmine and bougainvillea scaled wooden supports to the eaves, then stretched up over the roof. It was as if nature had embraced this little house and made it her own.

"It's open," a voice called from inside.

I climbed the three steps to the porch and let myself in. The house smelled of antiques and fresh mint. After pausing a moment in the entryway to get my bearings, I stepped into the living room. A vaulted ceiling rose to a roughly hewn exposed beam. Strategically placed rugs of varying size protected the dark hardwood floor. Two Craftsman chairs and a matching couch sat in a semicircle facing a large stone fireplace that dominated the wall to my right. Oddly, the house felt much larger inside than it appeared from the outside.

To my left, a round wooden table and four high-backed chairs sat in a small dining area. Beyond that was the kitchen, where I found Nate.

He stood at the sink with his back to me.

"Sam?" he called over his shoulder.

"Yes, sir, hello."

"Take a seat. I'm making tea." He spoke in a rich, voice-of-God baritone that imbued even mundane words with gravitas. "Chamomile okay with you?"

"That's fine." I sat down at the table. On the wall in front of me, an oil painting of rolling hills and bent oaks hung between two sconces. It reminded me of the unspoiled landscapes I had admired on trips through the central California coast.

Nate appeared in the kitchen doorway holding two large, brown glazed mugs. He stood about five foot seven and looked to be in great shape for a man who was probably in his late sixties. A shock of wavy white, shoulder-length hair framed a tanned face with high cheekbones and a strong jaw—features that reflected Native American ancestry. He wore faded blue jeans, old work boots, and a red plaid flannel shirt with the sleeves rolled up to the elbows. His hand-tooled leather belt was fastened with a silver buckle that was a little large for my taste, but it looked fine on him. So did the whole outfit. Worn-in, honest clothes. Unlike my usual Hawaiian shirts and flip-flops.

"Have any trouble finding me?" he asked.

"Not a bit," I lied.

He sat down on the opposite side of the table and looked me over. "So, to what do I owe the pleasure of this visit?"

"I'm in the music business, a songwriter. And let me tell you, it's a bitch," I blurted with none of the usual pleasantries. "I've got a hit; people are finally paying attention, and I need to take advantage of that. But I'm empty. I couldn't write a tune to save my life—my mojo's gone AWOL!"

"Whoa, boy," Nate cut in. "Your career is *your* business. Mine is to get you in shape, so you can succeed at whatever you choose to do." He examined me. "I'll give you this: You're not exactly ready to take the world by storm. How old are you?

"Forty-one."

He motioned to me. "Come into the light and let me have a look at you."

I moved over to the seat next to his. He leaned uncomfortably close, then grabbed my chin and stared, first into my right eye and then the left, tilting my head back and forth, up and down. This went on for over a minute. The old man was so intent I almost burst out laughing.

Finally, he sat back and took a deep breath.

"I see blood sugar issues—if you don't feed yourself every few hours you'll keel over. Your energy is generally low, but even worse between two and four in the afternoon. And your mind is a beehive of activity. Bet you have a hard time falling asleep at night."

"Yes, I do."

"There's sinus and respiratory problems. It looks like you inherited allergies and bad lungs from your father."

"Yeah. I'm told he gave me his hay fever and asthma."

"And you can thank your mother's genes for your weak intestines."

"My mom's father died of colon cancer and her brother has had colitis for decades."

"Not surprising."

He tilted back in his chair. "Did I miss anything?"

"How do you know all that?"

"It was simple. Your eyes told me about you. So, you're forty-one."

"Uh-huh."

"But you feel sixty-one. Am I right?"

I nodded, still wondering how he performed that bit of magic. "Really, how *did* you —"

"Fatigue is very common among folks your age."

Clearly, the subject of wizardry was closed.

"Why is that?"

He clasped his hands behind his head. "Well, most humans are arrogant enough to think they're above the laws of nature. They push themselves to their bodies' limits. They eat what suits them instead of what serves them. They sleep too little and stress too much."

I started to respond, but Nate continued. "Up to thirty-five or so, you might not notice the damage you're doing. Nature considers you a very valuable commodity and uses all her powers to protect you from yourself. But beyond that you're on your own."

"I don't understand."

"Perpetuation of all Earth's species is one of her top priorities. As long as you can be of use in that department, she does everything she can to protect you, even if you neglect yourself. By the time you're in your mid-thirties, nature figures she's given you enough time to reproduce and raise your young. In other words, you've become dispensable. That's when you'll notice you can't get away with the same self-abuse without suffering consequences." He pointed to my gut. "Don't have much practice taking care of yourself, do you?"

My neck stiffened. "I do all right." Then I glanced at my bloated belly. "Okay, obviously there's room for improvement."

"Well," Nate said, "nature is always there for you. She doesn't judge or condemn. She's just a force—one to be reckoned with, for sure. Stay on her good side, abide by her rules, and all will be well."

I took a good look at the old man. He was uncommonly vibrant, and healthier looking than most of my friends. "If that's true, why don't more people do it?"

"Most folks aren't ready to take responsibility," he said matter-of-factly. "That would require them to do something about it. Old habits, even destructive ones, are comforting. Change is unsettling. People resist it no matter how bad off they are."

"I can't disagree with you about that," I told him. "But I know I need to change. Enough to answer your crazy ad."

He studied me intently as he considered his response. "Well, I can teach you what you need to know."

"Is this where you tell me it'll cost a small fortune?"

"Hell, I don't need your money," he said, waving off the question. "But later on, maybe we can find something you can do for me."

"Like what, write you a song? It's about all I know how to do." For the first time in my life, I felt ashamed of that.

"We'll find something," he assured me.

We finished our tea in silence—its warm, subtle sweetness tasted good to me—and I caught myself feeling a little envious of him. He wore his convictions like a comfortable old coat while I was a bundle of nerves and unanswered questions.

"Nate—before—when you looked in my eyes. That was an amazing diagnosis."

"Oh, please, I didn't diagnose anything. Medical doctors use that word when they find a disease in you. I identified the *potential* for disease, your body's predispositions. Knowing those, you can usually avoid disease."

"Avoid disease?"

"Son, you need to understand that *you* control the experience you have in this world. The fatigue, aches and pains and that ample belly of yours are your body's responses to the choices you've made. You noticed these things happening and maybe they bothered you—but evidently not enough to make you change your behavior. Why do you think you can't write a song anymore?"

I shrugged.

"Your body hasn't been able to get your attention any other way. It figured that if it dried up your creative flow, you might just wake up to what's at stake.

"Everything is connected, my boy," he added. "If you want your—what did you call it?—your mojo back, you'll need to learn to listen, and give your body what it needs."

He let that thought hang in the air for another moment.

"One thing is certain: Keep doing what you're doing and your condition will continue to deteriorate. You'll suffer decades of declining health and lost creativity until one disease or other finally puts you out of your misery. You can die a painful and premature death, if that's what you want." He bent forward. "Or maybe you'd rather have perfect health, live a hundred years, maybe longer. The choice is yours."

"I'm sorry, but that's hard to believe."

He reached across the table and touched my shoulder.

"You called me because you know you've got to make some changes. Right?"

I nodded.

"And deep down, you also know that if you don't make those changes, and make them soon, there's gonna be hell to pay."

He was hitting close to home.

"My boy, some part of you believes it or you wouldn't be sitting here."

He disappeared into the kitchen and remained there for several minutes, purposely I thought, to let his words sink in.

FOUR

Nate returned with a bowl of red grapes and set them on the table between us. He popped a few in his mouth and chewed for what seemed like an eternity. Finally, he spoke. "These are the last grapes till next summer. Have some."

"No, thanks."

"Suit yourself," he said. "Let's get back to the idea of avoiding disease. It's strange how many people believe good health is out of their control."

"Well, it's mostly genetics," I said.

"Not exactly," he said. "You inherit tendencies and pre-dispositions, but that's all they are." He reached behind me, took a length of chain off the sideboard and held it slack between his fists.

"This is you." He snapped the chain tight with agile hands. "Your genetic dispositions are like the links in this chain. Some are strong, some not so. If you don't take care of yourself," he snapped the chain again, "which links will break first?"

"The weak ones."

"Right! Ignore your weak links and you miss an incredible opportunity to take control of your health."

"Okay."

"But taking care of yourself involves more than understanding your own particular limitations. You'll need to learn the basic principles nature established that govern human existence."

"And you just happen to know all these basic principles?"

He let my sarcasm pass without comment. "You'll also have to understand the truth about the way things work in this world." He motioned to the window and the fog outside. "Unfortunately, that truth lies beyond a haze of misinformation."

Nate seemed like a down-to-earth guy, but this seemed a little grandiose.

"What kind of misinformation?" I pressed.

"Pretty much everything you've come to accept as fact—falsehoods whose roots are buried deep in the system man has created for himself."

"The system?"

"And the mass consciousness that perpetuates that system."

He returned the chain to the sideboard. "You will fail unless you break the grip mass consciousness has on you," he said, turning back to look directly at me.

"I have no idea what you're talking about."

"I'm talking about the unconscious, collective belief that keeps you and everybody else in line—predictable and uniform." He paused to see if he'd lost me yet.

"Go on."

"The system relies on unlimited growth and continuous expansion. It requires us to remain good consumers from birth to death and uses mass consciousness to keep us convinced that our life's purpose is to have all the things money can buy. If that means sacrificing our health, so be it."

Actually, Merry and I didn't care much about having stuff and keeping up appearances. We never had the money for it, not with *my* career. But I had to admit that I was driven when it came to wanting Zoë to have everything.

Nate planted his finger on my chest. "Taking care of this body demands time and energy. But there are only so many hours in a day, and 'wasting time' taking care of yourself doesn't jive with the system's priorities. So, you are led to believe that sleep is overrated, that a couple of workouts each week will keep you in shape, and that fast food is real food."

I was sure he could see me squirming.

"This ringing any bells?" he asked.

I wasn't going to volunteer that I hadn't exercised since high school.

Nate walked to the window and gazed out into the fog. "You watch TV? he asked.

"A little."

"In the early evening, ever notice how many commercials there are for pizza places, frozen dinners and snacks, what do they call 'em, convenience foods? They know you'll buy that stuff because you're too busy to take the time to eat right."

He turned to face me again, his features darkened by the eerily filtered light behind him. "Then later come the commercials selling you over-the-counter medicines for heartburn, gas, acid reflux, constipation, and diarrhea—which you're guaranteed to need if you eat the garbage they sold you earlier. And that suits the system fine."

At the mention of heartburn, the dull pain in the center of my chest began to throb, and the feeling intensified as Nate took off like a fire-and-brimstone preacher.

"When your body finally breaks down from the abuse, you graduate to become a reliable consumer of the system's prescription drug and medical establishments, convinced that medicine and surgery are your only options. Health care," Nate said, making quotation marks with his fingers, "is one of the system's most profitable sectors."

"Wait a minute. Are you saying that modern medicine is a sham?"

"Not at all," he said. "There's a real need in this world for skilled doctors. But human beings are not simply a collection of symptoms to be managed. We're a collection of behaviors and choices. Medical science will never reach its full potential until it recognizes that. They can throw all the money in the world into research, but they'll never find the truth in a double-blind, clinical study."

"How else are we supposed to learn the truth?"

A sly smile spread across his lips and his eyes narrowed. "We can *remember* it."

He sat down, reached into a drawer on his side of the table and pulled out a tiny, slide top wooden box. Something inside rattled as he handed it to me.

"What's this?" I asked.

"A little inspiration. Humans are naturally skeptical creatures, always needing proof before we can accept something. Take a dozen of these tonight before bed."

I stuffed the box in my jacket pocket. "Are these vitamins?"

"It's *real* food," he said. "In fact, it's the simplest and purest food on the planet." He reached into the drawer for an identical box, tapped a couple of small, green pills into his hand and tossed them into his mouth. Then he turned to me and spread his arms like Charlton Heston parting the Red Sea. "Until a man is convinced something exists, he cannot fully desire it. Before he will make an effort to acquire it, he must *believe* it can be obtained." He pointed at me and winked.

"You've got a lot of work ahead of you. The contents of that box should provide some motivation." He seemed more than confident. "You know, in a way, you've already succeeded."

"How's that?"

"Well, by following the wrong directions, you have successfully found your way to the Land of the Lost Mojo." He laughed at the joke and then became serious again. "To get where you *want* to go, you're gonna need new directions." He rose from his seat. "Now if you'll excuse me, I've also got work to do."

I stood up, disoriented. "Is that it?"

"For now."

"When should I see you again?"

"You'll know."

FIVE

I needed time to think, so I took the coast highway north through Malibu to Zuma Beach and sat for a long time, pushing sand through my toes, going over what Nate had said.

Better choices lead to a healthier, more balanced life— that *was* common sense. And, clearly, I needed to boost my energy, feel more creative and get back to work. But that business about "mass consciousness" and everyone being a consumer was a little hard to take. *How do you make a living without selling your goods or services or songs? And how do you sell them if no one is going to buy them?* I wasn't sure Nate really had that part figured out. But he'd definitely figured out something. The man was so *alive*. If my eyes were as clear as his, I could probably figure things out for myself, "haze of misinformation" or no.

I wanted to, but couldn't imagine how.

∾

At home, Merry and I packed Zoë—and what seemed like half her things—into the Volvo, a process so elaborate that it was close to sundown when we finally parked at Fourth and Arizona. We pushed the stroller onto the crowded sidewalk and walked to the Promenade, one block west.

Merry and I had put off having a baby for a few years after we married, and when we were finally ready, it took us another three years, and one miscarriage, to have Zoë. Our marriage barely survived the frustration and heartbreak. But now, walking with my new family, all I could feel was a warm, almost primordial sense of satisfaction.

I glanced over at Merry. Despite everything she had endured, she looked completely happy... and so beautiful. Wisps of soft, shoulder-length blond hair fell across her face—a great face with a creamy complexion that needed no makeup at all. And she'd regained her great figure.

"Nice night," is all I managed to say.

We made our way through the crowd, past the assorted collection of kiosks, vendors, artists, and street performers. A gleam caught my eye—the setting sun reflecting off the polished metal of an old-fashioned vendor's cart parked just ahead. A sign on the front read:

HOT CHESTNUTS
$1.00

"You hungry?" I asked Merry. She was checking the baby for the third time in as many minutes.

"No, thanks. I ate before you got home."

A juggler started to draw a crowd.

"Go ahead. I'll catch up with you."

I stepped up to the cart and found no one on the other side. A small card with scalloped edges sat on the counter. Printed in green ink were the words "Ring Bell for Service." That seemed like a ridiculous idea, given that no one appeared to be minding the cart; but I hadn't eaten since breakfast, and my hunger was getting the best of me. I tapped the bell once and looked around expectantly. No one came.

I began to feel dizzy, and a cold sweat broke on my skin. I clutched the cart to steady myself.

"Good evening," said a strong voice.

I looked up and found a tall, good-looking African American man behind the cart. He was middle-aged, and his complexion was the color of caramel. His pale blue eyes looked luminous in the fading light.

"Beautiful night isn't it, Sam?"

I straightened up, loosening my grip on the cart. "I'm sorry, what did you say?"

He pointed to the sign. "Not many people ring that bell this time of year. You must be a real fan." His smiling eyes seemed to wink without winking. "One bag?"

I nodded, handed him a dollar bill, and accepted a small white bag. I removed a nut and instantly started to feel better.

As my head cleared, I got a better look at the man. He wore charcoal gray slacks and a dark blue blazer that framed a crisp, powder blue shirt and a red and navy blue striped necktie. He held his hands behind him, which squared his shoulders, giving him a distinguished, almost noble air.

"I haven't had a roasted chestnut since I was a kid," I said, wedging my thumbnails into a crack in the shell to pry it open. The nutmeat was warm and soft, and its distinct aroma and sweet taste filled me with nostalgia.

"In the winter, my parents would take us to Central Park in New York City. I remember the chestnut man—he had a cart like yours. It's funny, one of my favorite childhood memories is sharing hot roasted chestnuts with my brothers and chasing them through the snow."

"In that case," said the vendor, reaching under the counter and producing another bag, "please accept this gift, from one nut lover to another. I hope they bring you many more good memories."

As I savored another nut, I realized how odd it was to find hot chestnuts, always a winter treat, for sale on a warm October day in Southern California.

I left the cart and continued my stroll along the Promenade.

The setting sun was tinting the clouds over the ocean shades of orange and purple, and the wind began to pick up. I noticed a shift in my state of awareness as all my senses sharpened.

This is *a beautiful evening.*

The temperature was perfect, and the soft air smoothed my face and bare arms. I took a deep breath—my body felt electric. Suddenly, I could feel myself running at dusk through the open fields that lay behind my childhood home in Westchester County. My legs, powered by boundless energy, propelled me up and down the narrow dirt paths that crisscrossed the surrounding hills. The wind rushing past my face made it easy to imagine that I wasn't running at all, but flying, as I swooped up and around with no effort. Racing home into the deepening twilight, I felt exhilarated, joyful, and full of life.

"Sam!" A distant voice called.

"Sam? Hello, are you there?"

It was Merry. We were standing in front of a kitchenware store. Evidently, she had been trying to get my attention for a while.

"Where have you been?"

"I just had the most powerful memory," I panted, still feeling a little breathless. "Remember how much energy you had as a kid?"

"Vaguely," she said.

"Do you ever wonder where all that energy went?"

"I know where *mine* went," Merry said, motioning to Zoë. She arched her back against both hands and let out a long groan. Then she added, "Maybe it's just a natural part of growing older."

"But what if it isn't? What if we were meant to feel energetic and healthy our whole lives? Think about it. Adult monkeys swing from treetops. Grown lions have no trouble chasing down zebras. Why would nature single out humans and doom them to decades of breaking down and falling apart?"

"You're so sexy when you get philosophical," Merry teased. "It's a mystery, all right." She turned to the window display, distracted by a set of blue and yellow dishes.

Just then I heard the rhythmic strumming of a twelve-string guitar. It was the introduction to Joni Mitchell's song "Big Yellow Taxi," played with the full sound and overtones that can only come from open tuning.

I followed the music to a young woman with long, blond hair. She wore a white cotton blouse over an ankle-length tie-dyed skirt. There was purity in her voice and an unspoiled quality about her that reminded me of college girls I had known in the late '60s. We'd been so optimistic then about changing the world.

When she got to the tag-line chorus, I knew at once why I was drawn there. She sang sweetly: "Don't it always seem to go that you don't know what you've got till it's gone?"

I leaned down to her guitar case and dropped in a dollar. A dollar for unpaved paradise and that little kid still running inside me.

∽

At home, Merry and I hardly spoke. She was busy with Zoë, whose "unopened chakras" had her fussing, and I was lost in thought. The day had seemed so bleak when I woke, but I felt surprisingly hopeful now. Nate. Chestnuts. A girl with a guitar. Somehow, things seemed possible. How little it took.

As I undressed for bed, I discovered the box of tablets Nate had given me. I counted out twelve, knocked them back two at a time and swallowed them with several gulps of water. They didn't kill him—I was up for a dare. Exhausted, I kissed both my girls and barely managed to crawl under the covers before falling into a deep sleep.

SIX

When I opened my eyes, morning light was beginning to drift into the bedroom. It was only 6:30, but for the first time in months, I felt rested, totally energized. Nothing hurt.

I hopped out of bed and into the shower, humming and whistling under the splashing water.

As I finished, there was a knock on the bathroom door.

"Sam," Merry called, sounding half asleep, "is everything okay?"

Naked and dripping, I swung open the door. "Better than okay. I can't remember the last time I felt this good!"

Merry looked me up and down approvingly. "You look pretty damn good, too."

We wasted no time in acting on the attraction that sparked between us, making love for the first time since Zoë's birth. Waves of pleasure swept through us, back and forth, until, finally, we lay still in joyful exhaustion.

"That was nice," Merry sighed. "Just tell me something."

"What's that?"

"Who are you and what've you done with my husband?"

"Very funny."

"No, really—what's gotten into you?"

"I'm not sure," I said. Then I remembered.

"Last night I took some pills I got from Nate, the guy I met with yesterday. He's into nutrition and other natural things. He said it was food."

Merry was already into her bathrobe. "Well, I'm not complaining about the results." She glanced at me over her shoulder and glided out of the room.

❧

Zoë obligingly slept in that morning, and we made the most of it, flirting like teenagers over bagels and coffee for the next half hour. Then, with the sounds of stirring in the nursery, Merry was gone.

"You've been restless lately," she called from the other room. "Maybe you should get back to work. Don't you have a project to finish up?"

Geoffrey and I had a side gig developing old material in the catalogs of a few publishers in town. We were reworking the Tommy James hit, "Crystal Blue Persuasion," with an R&B feel for Windswept Pacific, the publisher who owned the copyright.

"Oh, yeah. The vocals aren't finished yet."

"Sounds nice," she said. "Why don't you give him a call and work on it today."

I glanced at the clock. It was 7:30. Geoffrey wouldn't be awake for at least a couple of hours. So I holed up in my studio for another staring match with our stalled songs. In minutes I was in default mode again, finger-picking tunes by Bert Jansch, Dave Van Ronk, Elizabeth Cotton, and John Fahey. My old Martin guitar's tone had become rich and resonant over the years. Funny thing. It only got better with age. Maybe there was hope for me too.

A little after ten, I put down the guitar and checked in with Geoffrey. Naturally, I woke him.

"Sam—glad you called," he croaked. "Jonathan Stone at Windswept wants to pitch our version of 'Crystal Blue' to some group in England, and he needs a tape tomorrow."

"Do you have the singers lined up?" I asked.

"We're in my studio at noon today. Can you make it?"

"Sure," I said, thankful the production was nearly complete.

"Hey, Sam?"

I was positive Geoffrey sensed something.

"If I call it in, would you stop at Palermo's and pick up a couple of pizzas? I'm starving."

I agreed and hung up the phone.

The morning paper lay open on the kitchen table as I passed by on my way to the bedroom. Eight words in large, bold print occupied the center of an otherwise empty half page.

WARNING:
THE SYSTEM IS HAZARDOUS
TO YOUR HEALTH

"If you say so, Nate," I said out loud. "But at the moment, I'm feeling pretty damn good."

❧

It didn't last long. I was already fading as I left the house, and by the time I got on the eastbound Santa Monica Freeway, my energy had completely sagged. That sweet reprieve from my aches and pains was over too. I stopped for the pizzas and continued north on Vermont, toward Geoffrey's house in Los Feliz.

The smell of pepperoni and cheese from the backseat was a loud reminder that it had been five hours since breakfast, and I was feeling a little light-headed. The closer I got to Geoffrey's, the faster my mind raced.

How could I let him think I was close to having something we could pitch? It's one thing to lie to an A&R man, but Geoffrey's my brother. He's gonna be so pissed. I wouldn't blame him if he started looking for another writing partner.

The sound of shattering glass and grinding metal jolted me back into the car. I lurched forward against the seat belts as the Volvo's front left fender plunged into the driver's side door of the car in the opposing lane. I jammed my foot on the brake and cut the steering wheel to the right. But it was far too late for that. I kept shearing down the other car's left side, crushing its mirror, door handles and molding before tearing off the rear bumper.

We came to a stop in the middle of the intersection. A small group of people gathered. I got out of my car. Three small figures sat inside the damaged Honda Accord, two in the front seat, one in the back. They were kids—couldn't have been more than seventeen.

"I'm so sorry," I said, bending down to the driver's side window. "Is anybody hurt?"

"What the hell's the matter with you, man?" the driver shouted. "Are you blind?"

A surge of adrenaline made me jump back, and from that vantage, I got a good look at the car. It was maybe ten years old, but a few minutes ago, the old Honda had been in immaculate condition—even its paint job looked fresh.

"You have every right to be upset," I said, handing him my business card. "I'm just glad that none of you were hurt."

"Yeah," he said gloomily, as if that were small consolation. He stuffed the card into his shirt pocket. "My dad will call you."

We exchanged insurance information, the Honda limped away, and the crowd dispersed.

"They're okay," I assured myself. "They're all okay."

But I wasn't. If I'd veered even one foot farther to the left, there would have been a head-on collision. I could have killed myself and those kids. Merry might have been a widow…Zoë wouldn't have a dad.

I pulled to the curb to inspect my car. The left headlight and bumper were scraped and chipped, but that was the extent of the damage. I climbed into the rear seat, slid the disfigured pizzas back into their boxes and sat there, waiting for my body to stop shaking. Finally, I drove the remaining block and a half to the studio.

❦

The recording session was a near disaster. Normally, Geoffrey works the board and I coach the musicians and singers. I managed to get a reasonably good performance out of the lead singer, but I couldn't focus, and none of my ideas for the backing vocals worked. Geoffrey repeatedly had to jump out from behind the console to help me arrange the parts. Finally, sometime after three, we managed to cut a few tracks we could live with. Geoffrey wrote each singer a check and then we were alone.

"Look, Sam, I didn't want to say anything and put more pressure on you, but come on, man. You really blew it in there today. You stay this zoned out and we're both screwed. I've been holding it together, drumming up gigs for us. But we both have to be there for this to work. And you are not there, man. You haven't been there for months." He ran the back of his hand across his mouth. "How's that tune coming you were working on?"

"Yeah, well…about that…"

"Jesus Christ, people finally want to hear new songs from us, and all we can show them is the same old stuff. I watch you during those meetings and you don't even try to act like you care. I know you can't force it, but you're not even going through the motions." He paused to compose himself. "I don't think I can let you keep doing this."

"What can I say? I'm sorry."

"I don't understand you. We get on the map with this hit and, with that perfect timing of yours, you decide to have a little breakdown." He walked over to the window and stared outside. "I don't know. Maybe you need a break to get yourself together, go sort things out. Take a vacation. Find a guru. Take up juggling. Whatever you need to do."

I swallowed hard. "A little time off might be a good idea."

He took a deep breath and released it. "I can tell people you're in rehab for a few months. Just let me know when you're ready to get back to work, okay?"

I joined Geoffrey at the window, and we looked out on the street without talking for a long time. I didn't want to leave—it would seem too much like an ending. But eventually, we walked, arms over each other's shoulders, onto his wooden porch.

"Shit, man. You are such an idiot," he whispered, a genuine smile breaking through.

"I don't know what I'm going to do," I said. "Any other suggestions?"

Geoffrey turned and put his hands on my shoulders. "Just take good care of yourself. And keep in touch, will you?"

I could feel his eyes on me as I stepped off the curb and walked across the street to the car. The sight of the fresh scrapes flipped my stomach.

God, I feel like hell. I strained to position myself behind the wheel.

Through the car's open window I looked west, deep into the late afternoon sky. I needed to see Nate. But the sun was about to set, and I'd have to wait until morning.

SEVEN

The marine layer was extremely dense when I arrived at Nate's, but I charged into the woods and up the noisy gravel path toward the little house concealed in the mist at the top of the hill.

The front door was open. Through it I saw Nate balancing on his left leg in front of the glowing fireplace. His right leg was bent so his foot rested against the inside of the opposite thigh, and his palms were pressed together in front of his chest, as if in prayer.

Not wanting to disturb him, I stood quietly and watched.

After about a minute, he took a deep breath and opened his eyes.

"Good morning," he said softly.

"That's 'tree pose' isn't it?"

"That's right. Do you practice yoga?"

"No, my wife does, though."

"Good for her." He stepped out of the pose. "Do you think you can do this?"

I was no yogi, but balancing on one foot didn't look too hard. "No problem," I said, going straight into the pose, hardly wobbling.

"Now close your eyes."

I did, and immediately listed sideways and crashed onto the couch. I jumped up, rushing to regain my composure.

"Wow. How come you can do that and I can't?"

A stern look flashed on his face. "Because I don't need my eyes to tell me where I am in the world and you still do. Because when you close your eyes, you become disconnected from everything. When I close mine, I get connected. *That's* how come."

I felt my face flush.

Nate's look softened. "That's all right," he said. "When you get plugged back in, you'll have no trouble performing that little balancing act." He patted me on the back. "How about a cup of tea?" Before I could respond, he disappeared into the kitchen.

I spent the next few minutes staring into the fire, wondering how, and from what, I had managed to get "unplugged."

"Come, join me," Nate called from the dining room as he set a tray on the table. I stepped into the room and my eyes widened. On the tray was a plate with a donut and an apple. "Here you go," he said, holding the plate in front of me. "Had breakfast yet?"

"Well, sort of."

"Which one would you like?"

I reached for the donut but grabbed a handful of air as Nate snatched the plate away.

"Did you really think I would feed you this poison?"

"It's just a donut," I said.

He picked up the apple in one hand and the donut in the other. "One of these will cure you, the other will kill you. Until you can see that and feel it in your gut, you don't stand a chance of getting connected. Eating must be a conscious action, not a mindless reaction."

"You really think I'm ever gonna choose the apple?"

"At some point, this apple will become irresistible to you." He handed it to me.

"If you say so." I put the apple down.

We drank our tea and things got quiet.

Finally, I broke the silence. "I took those tablets you gave me."

"And?"

"I woke up feeling great."

His face brightened. "Sounds like nature gave you a glimpse."

"Of what?"

He looked at me for a long time as if he were sizing me up, making a decision. Then he stood and walked to the far side of the living room. I noticed how easily and gracefully he moved. He pulled a small, leather-bound notebook from a bookcase that stood against the far wall, paused, then returned to the other side of the table, holding it against his chest with both hands.

"Question," he said. "If you wanted to take a trip to a place you've never been, how would you find your way?"

"I'd get directions or use a map."

"So, with guidance you would have complete confidence in your ability to reach your destination?"

"Sure, if the information's accurate."

"Fine. Are you aware that you are taking a trip at this very moment?"

"Really, where am I going?"

He flashed a half-smile but continued in an intensely serious tone. "This trip is called Life. Between its start and finish, you'll find yourself at countless crossroads. Your decision to go one way or another will determine where you end up and whether or not you arrive in one piece."

"Directions for *that* trip would be nice," I admitted.

"Nice?" he bellowed. "They're an absolute necessity. Look at yourself. Do you think you would be so completely lost if you had access to that kind of information?"

I suddenly felt uneasy. "Are you telling me there really is such a thing?"

He placed the notebook on the table. Carved into its cover were the words, *The Way Back.* Judging from its condition, the book was very old and worn by regular use.

"To succeed, you must be willing to accept that truth isn't always obvious, and may even be invisible to you," he said, laying his hand on the book's cover. "There's a delicate structure, beyond the physical plane, that conducts the energy which flows within and between all living things. It's called the biofield."

Gently, he opened the notebook. "But my father had another name for it." Handwritten in the middle of the first page were the words:

THE FIELD OF LIFE

He fixed his eyes on mine. "Ready?"

I nodded, and Nate began to read from the notebook.

"Thousands of years before civilization, humans shared the Earth with all the other life-forms, content with our place in nature's design. Back then, we possessed an ability that may seem fantastic, but is still common in what we now call 'the wild.' This ability enabled us to access a most wondrous creation, the Field of Life. The Field guided us through the natural world. It nourished and sustained us.

"But over time, humans grew tired of wandering the planet. We moved off the land and into cities of stone, abandoning the life nature meant for us, and we isolated ourselves from the natural order of things. But disconnection from the natural world came at a steep price. Over time, the Field became invisible to us, and we lost the ability to receive nature's guidance."

Nate took a sip of tea and then continued.

"Until recently, I, too, was unaware of the Field's existence. My life was dictated by man-made forces—jobs, clocks, money, and status. Then one day, I stumbled upon a combination of actions that reconnected me to this living fabric that organizes life on Earth. Instantly, my veil of ignorance lifted and the Field reappeared, stretching out in every direction.

"In that moment, the world became a new and miraculous place. My life since has been a grand adventure, exploring nature's treasures. I have recovered the vitality of my youth, and every day I am more and more alive."

Nate looked up to make sure he had my full attention and then continued reading.

"I expect these words will be dismissed as the ramblings of a man gone mad. Let me assure you they are not. For unless humans return to their proper place in nature's design, we put ourselves, indeed our entire planet, in grave danger.

"And so," he concluded, "I put pen to paper in the hope that sharing what I know may someday help others find their way back, before it is too late."

Nate turned the page, placed the open notebook on the table and walked into the living room to tend the fire.

"What did your father mean when he said 'before it's too late'?" I called across the room. "It sounds so apocalyptic."

"We'll get to that," he replied without looking up from the logs he was prodding.

My eyes fell onto the notebook and I read:

HOW IT WORKS

I reached over to turn the page.

"Please don't," Nate commanded from the other room. "The next lesson will begin in a minute."

EIGHT

"Fog's taking its sweet time lifting this morning," Nate said, slipping on a cable-knit wool sweater he retrieved from another room.

I checked the window and could barely make out the eucalyptus trees that stood just a few feet from the house.

Nate rubbed his hands together to generate heat. "You comfortable?"

"I'm okay," I said. Even with my jacket on, I was a bit chilly. But my curiosity outweighed my slight discomfort. "Nate," I asked, "this 'biofield'—can people see it?"

"Some can. But whether you see the Field of Life or not isn't important. What matters is that you're aware of it and understand its importance. One thing's certain, though—you won't see it until you're ready."

He turned to adjust the painting of bent oaks on the wall. "Sam, the ad that led you to me—had you seen it before?"

"No, why?"

"How often do you read the newspaper?"

"Every day."

"And you'd never seen my message before?"

"No," I insisted. "What are you getting at?"

He turned toward me.

"The ad's been running for quite a while. You only saw it when you were ready to change. Up to that point it was invisible to you because it would have made no sense for us to get together."

My thoughts swirled. "How long has it been there?"

"Long enough." He looked back at the painting and finished buttoning his sweater.

"Now, in my experience," he continued, "it's generally a good idea to know exactly what you're looking for before you go rushing off to find it." He picked up the notebook in one hand and grabbed his mug of tea. "It's still a little chilly. Let's move over by the fire."

He settled into the Craftsman chair to the right of the hearth. I sat on the couch. The flames cast a warm glow into the room. Nate grabbed an apple out of a bowl on the coffee table and tossed it to me.

"Here, feed your brain. I need you fully conscious for this."

I polished the apple on my shirt and took a bite.

For the next hour, Nate read aloud from the notebook. The information was very technical, very detailed, shifting from biology to physical science. I had to stop him repeatedly to ask questions. Now and then he would close the book, leaving one finger to hold his place, and paraphrase an especially dense section. He was a patient teacher, often going over a point several times from different angles, until he was satisfied I understood. Finally, he snapped the book closed and laid it on his lap.

"All right then," he said, "tell me about nature's Field of Life."

My heart jumped into my throat.

Nate laughed. "Relax." He got out of his chair and sat cross-legged on the floor. "Just tell me what you know about it in simple English, like I'm a child."

I froze, feeling like this was a pop quiz and I wasn't sure I'd done the homework.

"Look," Nate said softly, "I need to be sure that you have a grasp of the Field's basic structure. Otherwise nothing else I have to teach you is going to make any sense."

I took a deep breath. "Okay, if I understand you, the biofield is an incredibly delicate network of energy that covers the Earth. It stores, organizes and transmits that energy throughout the natural world, right?"

"The biofield actually extends far beyond Earth. But go on."

"You know, this 'Field' sounds an awful lot like the electrical power grid the Birkenstock types are always threatening to get off."

The old man's face turned to stone. "Hell, the two couldn't be less alike. Nature's biofield exists to safeguard Earth's resources, man's power grid destroys them. Hers sustains the fragile balance that permits life here, man's undermines that balance. Nature's serves every form of life, man's benefits only man. Hers is perpetual, ours is unsustainable."

"Okay. Got it."

"Good." He lowered his head. "Now close your eyes."

I shut them.

"Do you feel the warmth of the fire on your skin?"

"Yes." The sensation reminded me of sunbathing on Jones Beach as a kid.

"Imagine what you're feeling is the warmth of the sun. It is, in fact, the sun's energy, trapped in wood and released by fire. For a moment, think of what life on Earth would be like without that energy."

I pictured a dark, cold rock. "It's impossible. Without the sun there wouldn't be any life."

"That's right. The sun is the source of all life on Earth. But its rays provide more than daylight. They are the source of the energy that flows through the Field here on Earth."

"Yes, I see that."

"Good," he said. "Tell me more."

"Well, millions of years ago, just as the simplest life-forms were about to appear, nature laid out the biofield to support that life."

"And?"

"Through it, the sun's energy was transmitted into microscopic, single-celled plants that were able to use sunlight directly as fuel." The gears that had been turning in my mind finally clicked into place.

"That's what the green tablets are made of, isn't it?"

"Very good. The plant's scientific name is aphanizomenon flos-aquae—commonly known as blue-green algae."

"Algae?" I barked. "You fed me pond scum?"

"Call it what you like," he replied calmly, "that little miracle's special talent is combining sunlight with a few gases and minerals to create Life Force out of thin air. When you ate the algae, that Life Force was transferred to you."

Life Force. Its name was a perfect match for the "oomph" I had felt. My mind skipped from the little green pills to that amazing romp with Merry.

"What happened next?" Nate asked.

"What?" It took me a few seconds to realize what he was asking. "Oh! Okay, so, let's see..." I refocused as quickly as I could. "Once sunlight had been converted into a more accessible form of energy—what you're calling Life Force—the biofield was able to support more complex organisms. Over time, that Life Force was transmitted from the smallest living things to larger ones. This went on until the energy carried within the Field became concentrated enough to support creatures with the greatest needs for energy."

"And that, dear boy, is why man arrived so late to the party," Nate chuckled.

"But haven't I just described the food chain?"

"The food chain is only one manifestation of the Field that we can observe through our five senses," Nate said. "It's a reflection of the Field as it organizes Earth's life-forms into a balanced and sustainable arrangement. Each life-form has its special place and makes a unique contribution to the living energy that flows through it. Each is acutely aware of the interconnection of all living things, and each possesses an innate understanding of its shared dependence on the Field for survival."

"You mean ecosystems?"

"Not exactly. When man observes nature's ecosystems, he's using limited perception—only viewing the Field's effects, not the Field itself. See the difference?"

He didn't wait for my response.

"To find the truth, you must be willing to see the world as it is, beyond the man-made illusion you have mistaken for reality. Only then will you be able to align yourself with nature's design and live an authentic and balanced life."

Nate suddenly looked much older. "You wanted to know what my father meant when he wrote that man must return to his rightful place before it's too late. When we turned our back on nature, we lost all sense of natural order and knowledge of the workings of the world." He was somber, starting slowly but picking up speed as he went.

"Soon we had more questions than answers. We filled that void by creating our own order and placing ourselves in an exalted position, above every other life-form. Our ignorance fueled our arrogance, and we laid claim to the Earth. In the name of 'progress' we plundered her resources and decimated entire populations of plants and animals that stood in our way."

A queasy feeling came over me.

"Just look around," Nate continued. "Man is destroying nature's biofield. Each time we clear a forest, pollute a river, or drive another species to extinction, we weaken the living fabric that supports life on this planet. Now that fabric is threatening to tear wide open. If that happens, the consequences will be catastrophic."

"How can you be sure?"

"Because it happened before, sixty-five million years ago when a giant meteor struck the Earth. The impact sent a thick cloud of dust and ash into the atmosphere, blocking the sun's rays, cutting power to the Field. When the flow of Life Force slowed to a trickle, thousands of species of plants and animals perished."

"*That's* why the dinosaurs became extinct?"

"All the higher life-forms were lost. But creatures with the greatest energetic needs, like dinosaurs, would have been the first to go. Today that distinction belongs to man.

"Human activity accounts for half the energy used on Earth. From the moment we walked away from nature, we've thought of nothing but dominating this planet—and we've succeeded. It's ironic, don't you think? Our great success could prove to be our undoing." His attention drifted out the living room window.

"Nate, you're scaring the hell out of me."

"You're right to be afraid," he replied casually. "But what are you going to do with that fear? The way I see it, you've got only two choices: do nothing or take a stand."

"Take a stand? But there are billions of people on the planet."

"Don't underestimate the power of one person." He picked himself up and eased back into the chair. "When a body is sick, it doesn't heal all at once; it heals one cell at a time. The same is true for a sick planet. It too can heal—one enlightened person at a time. Learn the lessons I have to teach you, heal yourself and heal your planet."

I couldn't even write a song. Healing the planet was a bit of a reach. "You're talking to the wrong guy," I said. "You need Superman."

"Well, it's your choice," he said. "But consider this— putting yourself back in shape won't matter one bit if the planet becomes uninhabitable." He looked me straight in the eye. "I told you before that I didn't need your money. But this knowledge comes at a price. When people are shown the truth they have a responsibility to enlighten others."

"Right. But, realistically, how am I supposed to do that?"

"Each person finds a way. When the time comes, you'll know."

I shook my head. My mind was shutting down from overload. "No offense, but people are going to think I'm a nut if I go on about this."

Nate shrugged. "You'll find a way to do what you need to. And I imagine you'll do it the same way as everyone else I've taught."

"How's that?"

"Step by step, son. Step by step." He stood and quickly walked past me, through the dining room and into the kitchen.

"Nate?" I caught up with him as he headed out the back door. But before I could say another word, the view took my breath away.

NINE

The fog had lifted, and I found myself standing at the highest point visible for miles: a vast garden, webbed with dirt pathways, spread across the hilltop that was Nate's backyard. Its lush vegetation stood in sharp contrast to the dry, scrub-covered hills. Beyond the garden lay a panoramic view of the Pacific coastline, stretching from the Santa Monica Pier north to Malibu. Far in the distance, the ocean shaded into the sky.

"Welcome to my supermarket," Nate said. He grabbed a burlap sack at the bottom of the stairs. "Come on, I'll give you a tour."

He pointed toward the south end of the property. "Over here are the vegetables."

Giant sunflowers loomed above us as we made our way into the garden, and I stopped to admire the towering plants.

"Their dried seeds are good snacks. But I have to keep these monsters on the north side or they'll hog all the sunlight."

We walked past row after row of vegetables in various stages of growth. Nate pointed out the wispy tops of carrots, the elongated heads of romaine lettuce, the tomato vines trained to their stakes.

"Cucumbers like a little shade, so I plant them just east of the corn." Nate collected a handful of fallen leaves, stuck them in the burlap bag and slung the sack over his shoulder. "I'll show you the orchard."

I followed him down a rock-lined path that led across a small open area directly behind the house. We entered the orchard under a canopy of blossoms and were greeted by wafts of heady scents, birdsong, and the drone of bees. Some of the trees were in full flower, while others were ripe with fruit. Nate introduced me to a few of them by name: Hachiya persimmon, Shanghai peach, Desert Dawn nectarine, Santa Rosa plum, Fuerte avocado, Meyer lemon.

"There's no apple tree," I said.

"Not enough hours of chill at this elevation." Nate said. "The Fuji I offered you was from my friend's orchard in Tehachapi. At forty-two hundred feet above sea level, his apples ripen a good two weeks before anybody else's in this part of the country."

Nate plucked a tangerine from a low-hanging branch. "If you're going to stay awhile, you might as well make yourself useful." He pushed his thumb under the skin, which somehow fell off the fruit in one piece. Then he separated several wedges and handed me a few. "Come this way," he said, stashing the peel in his sack.

He led me to the back corner of the garden, where three large, open-ended wooden stalls stood side by side in the shade of a giant willow. The first was piled with freshly cut leaves, garden clippings, and kitchen scraps. The second contained matter that was slightly decomposed, and the last was filled to the top with a rich dark brown mixture. The stuff had an odd odor, sweet and musty.

"Is this compost?" I asked.

"Yup. Nature wastes nothing. I try to do the same."

Nate handed me a pair of garden gloves and pointed to an old wheelbarrow and shovel. "I'm getting ready to plant my broccoli, cabbage, and cauliflower seedlings and I'll need this compost to feed the soil."

He told me to take everything in the last stall up to the vegetable garden and pile it next to an unplanted patch of ground. After that, he wanted me to move the slightly decomposed heap to the last stall and the newer stuff to the center bin.

I stared at the three enormous heaps and began to calculate how long it would take to finish.

Nate cleared his throat, loudly. "Get to it, you're burning daylight." He dropped the burlap bag and strode toward the house, whistling to himself.

The moist compost did not yield easily to the shovel, and the loaded wheelbarrow was unwieldy. At first, I careened all over the narrow dirt path that led to the garden. My arms and legs tired quickly; my back and shoulders ached.

The job took all morning. Exhausted, filthy, and soaked through with sweat, I dumped the last load, laid the gloves and shovel in the wheelbarrow and dragged myself up to the house.

"Sam," Nate called from the kitchen window, "I'm making lunch. There's leaf lettuce growing between the rows of corn. Would you bring some in?"

I took a spade off a potting table under the stairs, found the lettuce hiding in the corn and wrestled the largest head out of the ground. When I handed it to Nate, dirt-laden root and all, he rolled his eyes.

"We harvest lettuce *above* the ground," he said. He made a sawing motion across the base of the plant. Then he tossed me a white towel. "You can use the sink behind you to wash up."

༄

The salad Nate prepared was a jumble of colorful vegetables. He set it on the table next to a tureen of split pea soup.

"Color matters," he said, serving me and then himself. "Each one has something special to offer the body. Green and yellow foods build and cleanse. Red foods stimulate. Blue and purple are healing."

Next to this meal, the canned, packaged and fast foods I'd been living on seemed dead as cardboard.

"The more live food you eat, the more alive you feel," Nate said. Then he sat back in his chair, closed his eyes and became very still.

I wondered if he could hear my stomach growling.

To hell with good manners, I'm starving.

I dipped my spoon in the soup and brought it toward my mouth. It was tantalizingly close when Nate opened his eyes.

"If you're hungry, you'll want to get the most out of this meal. Are you interested in a lesson?"

"As long as it involves eating," I said, returning the spoon to the bowl.

"You'll need to follow my instructions to the letter, all right?"

"I'll try."

"There will be no talking. You and I are going to eat in complete silence. Before you pick up the silverware, take a moment to truly appreciate this food, its colors and aroma. Take a bite and register its taste before you begin to chew. And chew thoroughly. Your body has only one set of teeth and they're not in your stomach. Swallow and sense the food moving inside to nourish you. Only then should you take another bite. When your stomach tells you that you've eaten enough, stop." With that, he began to eat.

The guy was a bit of a control freak, and I wasn't quite sure why I was submitting to all this. But I did. At first, the whole process of seeing, smelling, tasting and feeling was laborious and frustrating. I fought the urge to gulp the soup and down the salad in unchewed chunks. But after a few minutes of unhurried and deliberate eating, I began to really enjoy the meal—its freshness and the variety of its flavors and textures. It turned out Nate knew a lot about pleasure.

"How was that?" he asked, when he saw I was finished.

"Delicious."

"Anything else?"

"I feel great—satisfied, but not stuffed."

"Exactly," he said. "What you feel is your reward for patient, conscious eating. It is one thing to eat, and another to receive. Mealtime must be a ritual that is respected and protected. But for most folks, eating has become an afterthought. They eat on the run or in front of the television."

"That's me, all right."

"Eating has to be a conscious action. Intention is everything. When you sit down to eat, your intention must be to receive what the food has to offer you. Multitasking at mealtime is silly and dangerous. Would you ever consider driving your car and balancing your checkbook at the same time?"

"Of course not, but I don't have any trouble watching television or reading a book while I'm eating."

"Intention. Dictates. Outcome," he said. "If your intention is focused on watching television or reading a book, that's what you'll accomplish. But, I guarantee, you won't digest much. At mealtime, your conscious intention must be to receive what the food has to offer or you will absorb only a small fraction of the nutrients the body needs. And keep in mind," he added, pointing to my gut, "a malnourished person tends to overeat."

Nate stood and collected the plates. "Help me with these dishes and we'll get back to work."

When we headed out to the garden, he gestured to my gloves and shovel and led me to the pile of compost I had dumped.

"Spread the fertilizer a couple of inches thick," he said. "Then we'll fold it into the soil."

He made himself comfortable on an old gray teak bench and opened a pocket knife. Then he glared back at me. "Well?"

I was at it for more than an hour. I'd look over periodically to see Nate whittling an ever-shortening twig and wondered if that fantastic story about the biofield and our imminent demise was a ploy to get me to do his chores. As I finished, he looked up.

"What are you doing here?" he asked.

"Your work."

"Let me rephrase that. What exactly do you hope to accomplish?"

"I just wanted to feel better so I can get back to writing songs. Now it looks like I'm going to have to save the planet. Any idea when we'll get around to that?"

Nate continued whittling. After a moment, he shifted from the middle to the left side of the bench, which I took as an invitation to join him. We sat quietly for the next few minutes. Nate seemed content to pare away his stick. I was glad for the rest. Finally he set the twig and knife down at his side.

"Tell me how you write a song," he said. "With all the possible combinations of notes and chords, how do you decide which ones to use?"

I couldn't imagine why songwriting would interest him but decided to play along. "For me, a song is a picture painted with sound. My brother and I write together. So usually I start with lyrics he gives me that convey a specific feeling. Then I experiment with the changes, melody, and tempo until I find music that matches that feeling. When the song is finished, the words and music should sound like they were destined for each other."

"You say you experiment with the changes?"

"The chords. Musicians refer to chords as changes."

"Uh-huh. That's interesting. So, would you say that, to some degree, songwriting is a process of elimination?"

"Partly. Yes, I suppose so."

"I'm curious. How do you decide what to keep and what to throw away?"

My mind went blank. I hadn't posed the question to myself that way before. "After a while you just develop an instinct for it," I said finally.

Nate prodded. "So, you're here because you want to feel good."

"That's right."

"If 'feel good' was the name of a song, what do you suppose the lyrics would be?"

"I don't know."

"Oh, but you must. Designing a life is exactly like writing a song. But in this case, the lyrics describe your vision of how you want to feel, what you want to accomplish. The chords, melody and tempo are the various behaviors you'd experiment with until you found the ones that match that vision." He folded the pocket knife. "Feeling good won't happen by magic. Just as the lyrics inform the music, the vision determines the behavior."

"So the vision is something like what Geoffrey gives me—the story. You want me to write my own story?"

"That's one way of putting it," he said. "To bring that story to life, you'll need to remove the actions that don't serve it and replace them with others that do." He handed me the twig, smoothed of its rough edges. "But, you must know exactly what you want, and have a clear vision of the story you want to create, before you can know how to act."

I stared at the twig in my hand and shook my head. It's one thing to put a song together. A life is a few orders of magnitude more complicated.

Doubt must've been all over my face, but Nate offered scant comfort. "Guess you're gonna have to develop an instinct for it," he said.

He stood, grabbed the hoe at the side of the bench and began to fold the compost into the soil. "Go home," he said without looking up. "Come back when you can tell me what you want. Remember, lyrics first, *then* the music."

TEN

I wanted to believe that I possessed the kind of power Nate thought I had, but 41 years of living hadn't given me any real evidence of that. Rebuild my life from scratch? As I descended the gravel path into the canyon below Nate's property, I wondered if I had it in me to change and to really stick with it.

Turning south on the coast highway, I had a moment of clarity about at least one thing that would make me happy: getting home. I drove fast.

The house was quiet when I arrived, and when I checked the master bedroom, I found Merry and Zoë asleep, the baby nestled inside Merry's outstretched arm.

They were so beautiful, so vulnerable as they lay there. I couldn't imagine leaving them unprotected, or letting any-thing harm them, ever. No one was asking me to chase off wild beasts, thank God, but at the bare minimum, I could stay healthy enough to be there for them when they needed me.

I lay down, placed my hand on the small curve of Zoë's head and studied her sweet face. She could draw my attention to the here and now better than any other force on Earth. I'd been trying to do that for years. But until Zoë was born, I spent most of my time lost in the future or fretting about the past. Now, under her influence, I was staying present more and more.

When my mind returned to Nate's questions about what I wanted to accomplish and what my new, improved life would look like, it didn't flit away. My daughter was working her magic, even as she slept, and worries dissolved in her soft glow.

A musty, sweet odor filled my nostrils, and everything went dark. I brought both hands to my face. Why was I wearing garden gloves? I peeked between my fingers to see an endless row of self-propelled wheelbarrows heading toward me, swaying like drunks under their steaming loads. I turned. Behind me, dozens of shovels dove, one after another, into a mountain of compost and then re-emerged to fling their contents onto the staggering barrows. I tried to run but with each step, I sank farther into the layers of soft decay. I twisted and turned to free myself, as drunken wheelbarrows and dancing shovels wove across the undulating surface.

I grabbed hold of something solid—the leg of an old teak bench. On it, Nate sat conducting the chaos, slashing the air with a pocket knife he used as a baton. He glanced down at me and shook his head. Then he set the knife to a gnarled tree branch and disappeared in a blizzard of wood shavings.

I lost my grip, took one last gulp of air and went under. *What's that ringing?*

I held my breath and swam furiously through the darkness toward the sound. More ringing. I thrust upward with all my might, breaking through the surface just in time to gasp for air.

ᘐᕰ

"Sam, it's for you."

"Huh...who?" I opened my eyes to pitch-blackness.

"It's Geoffrey on the phone," Merry whispered, switching on a lamp.

I crawled out of bed, taking care not to wake Zoë, and stumbled into the kitchen.

"Hey, what's up?" I mumbled into the phone.

He sounded frazzled. "I've got two jingles that have to be delivered tomorrow, and I only have time to produce one of them. Could you handle the other one?"

"*Jingles?*"

"I've already written it. All you have to do is show up, arrange the parts, and mix it. We're talking about thirty seconds of music."

"Okay," I sighed. "What's the address?"

He gave me the address of a recording studio in Burbank he had booked the next day from ten to two. I assured him I'd take care of everything.

ᘐᕰ

The next morning Zoë slept in. Merry and I had a quick breakfast of toaster waffles and coffee, straightened the house, washed the dishes, and folded laundry.

"I'm glad to see you and Geoffrey back together," she said, handing me a sock.

"Let's just say it's a momentary truce," I said. "I'm glad to pitch in."

As we finished, I told her how guilty I felt about spending so much time with Nate in Topanga, away from her and the baby.

"You're exploring, honey. Isn't that the natural order of things?" she asked. "You go after big game, I take care of the cave and offspring." She leaned in for a kiss. Affecting a Katherine Hepburn accent, she cooed, "Happy hunting, darling. Do bring home something wonderful, won't you?"

I checked the time—it was 9:15.

"Jesus, I'm late." With no time to change from my T-shirt and jeans, I threw on a pair of sneakers and dashed out of the house.

∽

In the recording business, time is literally money, and there is no greater sin than showing up late for a session. So I knew I was in trouble when I saw the traffic. It was stop-and-go on both the 405 and 101 freeways, turning what should have been a 30-minute trip into a 45-minute slog. When I finally arrived at the studio, it was exactly 10 o'clock. My stomach was churning.

The receptionist showed me to Studio C, where I found the keyboard player, bass player, and drummer setting up their equipment. Through the control room window, a woman in a tailored blue suit was motioning for me to join her. I took a deep breath and walked through the insulated door.

"Good morning," I said, extending my hand to introduce myself.

"Geoffrey," she whined, "we have a small problem." Her nasal voice was distinctly non-musical. Given that we already had a problem, I saw no reason to bother her with the minor detail that I wasn't Geoffrey.

"I've been listening to your demo and I feel that it sounds...well...too young."

Too young? It was a Barbie commercial, for Christ's sake.

"Let's listen to it, shall we?" I said.

The track was light and bouncy. The tune was catchy. Geoffrey had done a good job. After several minutes of discussion, I persuaded the blue suit that beefing up the arrangement with electric guitar would be the best way to solve her "young" problem.

"Now if you'll excuse me," I said, "I'll see if I can find us a player."

I grabbed a handful of M&M's from a bowl on the console and began to work through the list of guitar players in my address book. After several calls, and a few more handfuls of candy, I got hold of a guy who could do the session but wasn't available until one. By the time I rearranged the track, worked out the parts with the players and recorded the rhythm section, the suit's small problem had set the production schedule back over an hour.

We finished cutting the vocal at 12:30. Fortunately, the singer nailed it on the very first take.

I pressed the talk-back button. "That was great," I said. "Hold on and I'll see if we need any overdubs."

"Excuse me...Geoffrey." It was the suit talking. Something about the vocal bothered her, something it seemed she was incapable of articulating. As she blathered on, I thought about Nate and how I wouldn't be seeing him again until I could figure out what I wanted in my life. That could take awhile. At that moment, all I could think of were things I didn't want. Dealing with clueless people like this woman topped that list.

Her mouth stopped moving.

"It's your dime," I said. "If you're not happy, we'll try it again."

We blew another half-hour laying down inferior tracks as the life oozed out of the vocal. Finally the suit said, "I don't know. What do you think?"

I think it's one o'clock and you've wasted enough time. I pulled up the singer's very first take, added a little EQ and chamber and played it back hot in the mix.

"How's this?" I asked.

"Yes," she declared, "that's the one."

The engineer rolled his eyes and quickly abandoned the mixing console.

The guitarist arrived. At the same moment, the keyboard player returned with food from a nearby taco stand. When you're on the clock in the studio, there's no such thing as a lunch break.

"I got you a bean and chicken burrito," he said, setting everything down.

Stressed out and beyond hungry, I dove into the take-out bag. In the five minutes it took the engineer to get sound on the guitar, I wolfed down the burrito, a bag of chips and a soda.

A half-hour later, the track was complete—and I was in agony. The burrito was burning a hole in my gut, and I felt like I was going to be sick. The cramped control room felt suffocating, but I'd have to tough it out till we were done.

Mercifully, the mix went quickly and at two o'clock sharp, I handed the master tape to the blue suit.

"Geoffrey, I love it. I think the session went very well," she said in a tone drenched in self-satisfaction. "We'll do this again real soon."

Not in my lifetime, I wanted to say. But this wasn't my gig to short circuit. I managed a smile, shook the woman's hand and got the hell out of there.

Nausea struck the instant I hit daylight. I raced to a trash bin at the end of the parking lot and up everything came—the breakfast waffles, the M&M's, the entire greasy lunch. I collapsed onto the pavement. The flies buzzed over the stink of garbage, and I felt like road kill. But, for once, I made the connection: I'd asked for this.

ELEVEN

I'd gotten a good look at the face of toxic. Toxic sucked it up for the nitpickers in blue suits and self-medicated with M&M's and belly-bomb burritos. That was no real revelation, but it sure was dramatic to see my "old and unimproved" self in action.

I could do better.

That night, I managed to corral my cynicism long enough to put into words what I really wanted. The future me would be healthy: trim, energetic, and pain-free. I would honor my body and respect its limitations. I would trust my feelings and express them freely, without fear. The new me would look forward to every day, successfully balancing work and play, parenthood and marriage. I'd be conscious, not sleepwalking. I'd be passionately in charge of my health—and my life.

Gathering every bit of inspiration I could muster, I summoned up a vision of this vital, vibrant "me," and committed it to memory. Then, batting back the urge to mock myself for having such basic desires, I wrote it down.

∞

When I arrived at Nate's the next morning, he was watering the plants on his front porch. He pointed to the wish list in my hand.

"What do you have there?" he asked.

"This is what I want," I said, offering him the page.

He took it and set himself down in one of the porch's two rocking chairs. I took the other seat, and for the next few minutes, I soaked up the peaceful atmosphere. It was good to be back in Nate's world. The trees rustled high above and lulled me into a rare state of tranquility.

Finally, he spoke. "To succeed, your desire for change must be stronger than your resistance to change." His words dropped into my quieted mind, and I could feel them ripple.

I rubbed my still-tender stomach. "I'll do whatever it takes."

He folded the paper and slipped it into his shirt pocket. "This vision, and your commitment to it, will simplify every decision you make from now on." Nate studied my face. "You look like hell. What happened?"

Reluctantly, I recounted the incident at the studio.

"That's what happens when you relinquish responsibility and allow circumstances to dictate your actions," Nate said.

I took a stab at defending myself. "A leisurely lunch, communing with my food would have been great. Unfortunately, I had work to do and didn't have that luxury."

Nate threw his head back and laughed. I noticed the man didn't have a single cavity in his mouth. "With all due respect, son, nature doesn't accept excuses. You got caught up in your own little agenda and forgot that she has one too."

He grabbed the watering can at his side and raised it over his head. "And her agenda always trumps yours." He tilted the can. Water streamed out the spout, down onto the wooden porch at my feet. "The love of gravity is the beginning of all wisdom," he said, keeping his eyes fixed on the miniature waterfall.

My brain struggled to decipher the words. "What do you mean?"

"Jump off a cliff if you want, but expect a messy landing. Nature's laws are immutable. Tip the full bucket, and the water spills, no matter how much you pretend it won't. A wise person comes to terms with that."

I looked at the puddle of water and then back at Nate. "Well, there's one thing I can't pretend away. Eating whatever I damn well please doesn't work anymore."

Nate nodded. "No one gets away with it." He fixed his eyes on mine. "If that episode at the studio taught you nothing more, it served its purpose."

As I met his intense stare, I knew there was no going back to my old, unhealthy lifestyle. But the idea of committing to something so … foreign to me made me nervous, and I could feel myself backing away.

I stood up, trying to break the spell. "What do you say I grab your father's notebook and we have another look at it?"

"Sam, sit. Be still. The information you want isn't in any book, and it's not up here," he said, tapping his right temple.

"Nature's messages for you are everywhere. Trouble is, you're in no condition to receive them."

"The more you talk, the more ignorant I feel."

He slapped both knees. "Now we're *getting* somewhere!"

"We are?"

"Absolutely! Admitting ignorance is highly underrated. In my opinion it's the only way to achieve true wisdom. Man's obsession with compiling information, measuring, testing, observing, comparing, and studying hasn't advanced our understanding of what really matters one lick." He frowned. "What do we have to show for all our knowledge? More disease, famine, war, and environmental devastation. If we humans have proven anything, it's that knowledge without wisdom can be a very dangerous thing."

I rubbed my aching head. "So what are we talking about?"

He reached over to an old portable radio that sat on a table between us. He flipped a switch, and soft classical music drifted into the air. "Does this radio have to know music in order to play Mozart?"

"Of course not."

"It only needs to receive the signal, right?"

I nodded.

"Nature never intended for man to know all her secrets. But just as this radio receives music, we can receive nature's messages—if we're tuned in."

"And when I get 'tuned in'?"

"Then, my young friend, you will understand the truth." He sat back in his rocker and surveyed the wooded scene in front of the house. A faint sadness swept across his face and lingered there for a moment. Then he was on his feet. "Right now I have a chore out back that could use another pair of hands."

৶৶

A couple of six-foot-long 4x4s lay on the ground at the bottom of the back steps. Nate handed me one, hoisted the other onto his shoulder and grabbed his tool kit and satchel. I followed him into the orchard carrying the post against my right thigh. My arms tired quickly, but I took a cue from the old man, shouldered the wood and found it much easier to manage.

We reached a wire mesh fence that separated the garden from the uncultivated hillside and followed it to the back of the orchard. About a hundred feet down the slope, two fence posts tilted precariously inward.

For the next couple of hours I helped Nate reset the old posts and install new ones next to each for added support. He went about his work like a nimble young craftsman, and I tried not to get in the way. When we finished, he stood at the fence and scanned the other side. "They almost made it through this time."

"Who are 'they'?"

"My goats," he said, pointing to the far side of the hill. At the edge of the ridge, two heads bobbed up and down in the tall grass.

Nate reached into his satchel and pulled out a couple of apples. "I'll introduce you." He held the apples above his head and gave a quick whistle. The goats instantly turned away from a bush they were dismantling and started toward us.

"Your goats come when you call them?"

"Don't yours?" he chuckled.

73

The buck arrived first. He was black with a white under-belly and stood about two-and-a-half feet tall. I sensed an aggressiveness about him that made me nervous.

"Sam, I'd like you to meet George." He reached over the fence and the goat snatched the apple out of his hand. Nate stroked the animal's sturdy side. "Care to pet him?"

"No, thanks."

Just then, the doe arrived. She was a gorgeous chocolate brown and slightly smaller than the male. There was a sweet, docile quality about her. It may have been my imagination, but she seemed more gracious, more appreciative, as she accepted her treat.

"This one's Gracie." Nate gave her his full attention, and the two shared a moment of affection. "This land and the goats enjoy a mutually beneficial relationship," Nate explained, stroking the nanny's neck. "The hill feeds the goats, and they keep it clear of weeds and brush. George and Gracie know that the garden is off limits, but it's in their nature to try to get in here.

"We humans like to think we can suppress nature, control it. But we're deluding ourselves." Nate stepped away from the fence and the goats wandered off. "In the end, nature will always prevail. So it's wise to look for ways to get along with her." He collected his gear. "And that's much easier to do when you're tuned in."

"Right, like a radio."

Nate started up the hill. "Except that, unlike a radio, you are a dynamic, protoplasmic entity, capable of receiving and trans-mitting an infinite number of signals on multiple frequencies."

"Of course," I said. "I was just about to say that."

TWELVE

I hurried up the hill and through the orchard, and found Nate sitting at a small, round-topped table in the yard behind the house. The table's pedestal and surprisingly comfortable seats were fashioned out of old tree trunks that had been stripped and finished to withstand the elements. As I sat across from him, he reached into his satchel.

"Time to test your powers of reception." He produced two more apples and lobbed one to me. I caught it left-handed, transferred it to my right hand and polished it against my shirtsleeve.

"Pass complete!" I flashed him a grin and took a bite.

Nate chortled. "Nice catch, Jerry Rice. But this is about another kind of reception. I'd like you to describe everything you are experiencing right now. Simply explore your field of awareness and tell me what you notice."

I looked around and began to describe the view: the beautiful garden and surrounding hilltops, boats on the ocean, passing clouds. When I exhausted the visual field, I concentrated on sounds around me: birdcalls, the creaking hinge of an unlatched gate, tinkling wind chimes. I took a bite of the apple and described its juicy taste: part tart, part sweet. The scent of blossoms caught my attention and I did my best to characterize their flowery aroma. I ran my hand across the tabletop and described the knots, niches and subtle undulations of its surface.

"That's about it," I said, certain I had covered everything.

"Very good," Nate declared, clapping his hands.

"Thank you, thank you." I bowed with a flourish.

"Yes, sir," he continued, "you have a real flair for the obvious."

I waited a second for the sting to subside. "What?"

"*That* was a magnificent display of limited perception."

"What was so limited about it?" I asked, defenses rising.

"Run-of-the-mill, first-level stuff." He polished his apple against his sleeve. "Messages on the first level of awareness are so obvious, you'd have to be severely handicapped to miss them." Nate quartered the apple with his pocket knife and savored a wedge. "However, I am relieved to know that you are in full possession of your senses," he added. "They can be marginally useful."

He cleaned the knife on his pant leg and pocketed it.

"Every choice we make in life is a response to the unspoken question, 'If I do this, will it keep me safe?'" he continued. "People ask themselves this question countless times a day and have done so for over a hundred thousand years. It's an important question. Our very survival often depends upon coming up with the right answer.

"I'll grant you," he continued, "seeing, hearing, tasting, touching, and smelling all provide useful short-term information—'Did I turn off the stove? Is it safe to cross this street?' But if people aspire to thrive and not merely survive, they need to distinguish between actions that guarantee their *long-term* safety and actions that could lead them to harm down the road. Tell me, with which of your five senses do you make those decisions?"

"That's not a fair question. We don't have a crystal ball to tell us how every action's gonna turn out. Life's full of uncertainties."

"Granted, you don't have complete control over your future. But if you take the attitude, 'Life's a crapshoot—I could be hit by a bus tomorrow,' it's easy to fall into the mistaken belief that you have no control at all."

"Who's to say life isn't a crapshoot?"

"How about the Surgeon General? He just reported that 80 percent of Americans die prematurely because of unhealthy lifestyles and lousy eating habits. In other words, the choices they make are killing them." Nate leaned forward and stabbed the air with an apple chunk. "So, I ask you again. Which of your five senses can you rely on to help you make those choices?"

I shrugged.

Nate made a zero with his thumb and forefinger. "Every one of them is short-sighted. The look, smell, texture, and taste of a donut can render that junk virtually irresistible. Not one of your senses is capable of warning you of the lethal effects it can have on your body."

"I like donuts. Don't you think 'lethal' is a bit strong?"

"A little junk once in a while probably won't hurt you. The body's resilient. It'll tolerate a certain amount of abuse."

"And another thing," I pressed, "if they're so bad for me, why do they taste so good?"

"Junk food manufacturers have made a science of disguising their lifeless fare with chemical flavorings, aromas, and coloring, specifically designed to fool the senses. But if you weren't so out of balance, you wouldn't have the urge to eat that stuff."

"I have to admit; sometimes I do crave a good donut."

"Cravings are not to be trusted. Giving in to them will only cause greater imbalance, greater disconnection from the highest frequencies of the Field."

"Oh of course, the invisible Field of Life. Tell me again how I'm supposed to find that."

"When you can know without thinking, dream without sleeping—then you'll be ready."

Great. Another riddle. "So now what?"

"Close your eyes," he said coolly. "What do you notice?"

"Sounds."

"What about the sounds?"

"There are more of them."

"More than you noticed with your eyes open?"

"Yes, more. Quieter ones I didn't hear before: insects buzzing, the wind in the garden and the orchard."

"Keeping your eyes closed, plug your ears and tell me what you notice."

I stuck a finger in each ear and felt my body trying to settle down. A twitch developed over my right eye.

"Stay with it," Nate encouraged. "Let your body adapt to the quiet."

After a moment, the twitch subsided. "I feel cool air flowing through my nostrils."

"What else?" he asked.

"That's it."

"Sam, there's more. Be still and wait."

As my mind adjusted to the absence of external input, I became aware of subtle sensations inside my body. "There's a pressure behind my forehead and against each temple," I reported. "It's not a headache exactly, more like the beginnings of one." I shifted my position on the seat. "My lower back hurts, and there's an ache in my right shoulder that's working its way into my neck." My belly rumbled and a burp sent acid into my throat. "I'm hungry, but my stomach's still a little queasy from what I ate yesterday at the studio."

I unplugged my ears and opened my eyes to see Nate's broad grin. "Welcome to the second level of awareness," he said. "In every conscious moment, your body is expressing itself, communicating its likes and dislikes. You take an action, and the body tells you how it feels about that action. But instead of words, it uses symptoms to speak to you."

"I must've really pissed it off yesterday."

"The body prefers to whisper. But if you're not listening, it will yell as loudly as necessary to get your attention."

The pressure in my head intensified. "Why are symptoms so negative?"

"There are plenty of positive ones, too. For instance, when you wake up refreshed from a good night's sleep or feel energized after a nutritious meal. Those symptoms are your body's way of encouraging you to repeat healthy behavior. On the other hand, your body uses negative symptoms, like fatigue and stomach pain, to discourage you from sleeping too little or eating too much."

The clouds in my head were gathering fast. I closed my eyes, and a sharp pain shot through my skull. "Nate, I hate to interrupt, but I've got a splitting headache. Could I get a cup of coffee and maybe a few aspirin?"

"Sorry, no coffee, no aspirin."

I lowered my head onto the table. In an instant, Nate was halfway up the stairs to the kitchen. "Wait here," he said.

Don't worry, I'm not going anywhere.

The next thing I knew, he had laid a hot compress on the back of my neck and was gently wrapping another around my head. Within seconds, warm, earthy vapors rose into my sinuses and the pain began to subside.

"What is this stuff?"

"An old Indian remedy. How do you feel?"

"Better, thanks."

"Miss your caffeine fix this morning?" he asked.

"I tried a cup of coffee but it didn't sit well. So I skipped breakfast and came right over."

"No food *and* no fix." Nate shook his head. "It's a wonder you lasted this long." He produced a bowl of what looked like vanilla pudding and set it in front of me.

"What's this?"

"Goat yogurt, compliments of Gracie."

"Thanks, but I don't like—"

"Eat it," he commanded.

I sniffed the bowl and took a small taste. It was creamy and slightly tangy. "This is good," I conceded.

"Good and good for you," he said like a pitchman. "In the future don't be so quick to suppress your symptoms with medicine. Allow your body to express itself so it can guide you toward right action. That headache wasn't a symptom of aspirin or caffeine deficiency any more than yesterday's stomachache was caused by a lack of Maalox."

"Maybe so, but taking that stuff sure helps."

"Helps you into an early grave, you mean." Nate put his hand to his chin. He seemed to be rummaging through his brain for something. "Question," he said. "What would you do if you were driving and your car's oil light began to flash?"

"I'd check the oil, obviously. And if it was low I'd add some."

"Yes, of course. But let's say you don't want to bother checking the oil and decide to bash out that pesky warning light with a hammer."

"That's ridiculous. My engine would burn up."

"Uh-huh. Suppose your body is sending you a warning symptom, like headache or heartburn. Is it wiser to check the behavior that caused the symptom or pop a pill to suppress it?"

"Well—"

"Taking medicine to block pain is no different than bashing out your car's oil light. Both 'solutions' ignore the problem, and both are ultimately disastrous for the machine."

Just then, the back door swung open.

"Has he given you the crossroads talk yet?"

I turned to see a young woman coming down the stairs.

"I was getting to that," Nate said. He stood and met her at the bottom step. They gave each other a hug.

"I know you," I said after a moment. "You were at the Promenade a few nights ago, singing, with a twelve-string."

She turned toward me, keeping one arm around Nate's shoulder.

"Who's your friend, Papa?" she asked.

"Heather, I'd like you to meet Sam."

Her pretty face looked kind. "How do you do?" she asked.

"Not all that well," I admitted, holding the compress to my neck. "But I'm working on it."

"Oh, I see." She stepped closer, holding me in her warm gaze. Her eyes seemed to have the same purity I had heard in her voice. "A new arrival, huh?"

This girl was half my age but, I sensed, quite a bit further along Nate's path.

"Well," she said softly, "it's good you're here. Papa'll set you straight."

"Is Nate your grandfather?" I whispered.

She let out a full, uninhibited laugh. "Did you hear that?"

"I heard, and no, we aren't related. Though she is thinking of adopting me." He moved back toward the table. "Heather, why don't you see what's ready for market. Sam and I need to get back to work."

To my surprise, she reached to remove my compress and gave me a quick, maternal kiss on the forehead. Her fresh scent—castile soap with a hint of patchouli oil—triggered a memory of a college girlfriend. She'd been a hippie, unlike me, and I'd been scared off by talk of living on a commune. But I still admired the way she'd wanted to save the planet from the corporations, and the way she talked about peace and love. It was a little naive, maybe, but there was a sanity about it too.

"Welcome back." Heather said, as if she had been reading my mind. Then she disappeared into the garden.

THIRTEEN

"That kid's something," Nate beamed.

"What's her story?" The question immediately felt too personal.

"Today she's harvesting vegetables and fruit to sell at the farmer's market. Can't eat it all myself, now can I?"

Until that moment, it hadn't occurred to me that Nate sold what he grew.

"Heather and I have a business arrangement," he continued. "I grow it, she harvests and sells it, and we split the profits."

"Is she in school?"

"She graduated Santa Monica High last spring, top of her class, and was headed for Stanford till she found her way here. Once she discovered nature's Field of Life, she decided to hold off going to college so she could, as she put it, get her hands dirty."

"Whoa! She's seen the Field? How long did it take her?"

"Not your concern. And remember, not every person who wants to see it can."

I stirred my yogurt. "So, what's the crossroads talk?"

Nate pulled my wish list from his shirt pocket and waved the folded page. "This vision of your future—what you want—this is the destination. Now that you're in touch with messages on the second level of awareness, you have the makings of a rudimentary guidance system to find your way from where you are to here."

"I thought you said I'd be using the Field as a guide."

"You will. Nature's Field of Life is the ultimate guidance system. Fortunately, seeing the Field is not a prerequisite for accessing its power. But you haven't been granted that access just yet." He unfolded the paper and placed it on the table in front of him. "Every step you take along life's path has the potential to move you closer to or further from here," he said, tapping the paper. "A crossroads is a point on the path where choices intersect and you have to decide to go one way or another. Do you follow?"

"So far, but how do the messages on the second level help me decide which way to go?"

"Your body is an extension of nature, and you can trust it to give you accurate feedback. Remember when I offered you the apple and the donut? At that moment you stood at a crossroads. If you had stopped to consider your decision, do you still think you would have chosen the donut?"

"I honestly don't know."

"Let's assume that you were truly unaware of the disparate qualities of the apple and the donut, and your senses directed you to eat the donut. How would you have been able to tell whether that choice brought you closer to or further from your goal?"

I thought for a moment. As much as I liked donuts, they always made me feel jittery and a little spacey. "My body would tell me," I said.

"There's hope for you yet, my boy." Nate patted my shoulder. "Whenever you reach a crossroads and are unclear of the direction to take, make your best guess, keeping your destination in mind, and wait for the body's response. If you've stepped in the right direction, your body will reward you with a feeling of well-being. However, if you've chosen incorrectly, a warning light will go on. This warning may be subtle—lightheadedness or an inexplicable foul mood. It could show up as a craving for sweets or starch. Or it might come in the form of a headache, stomachache, or sudden fatigue."

"What's the use of warnings after I've already made the mistake?"

"Not a mistake, a detour. Soon enough you'll arrive at another crossroads and face another choice. The decision to eat the donut was a mistake only if you learned nothing from it. Next time you reach a crossroads that involves a donut, you'll remember that first encounter and redeem yourself by choosing wisely."

"I'm guessing that this works for decisions that are a little bigger than whether or not to eat a donut."

"Navigating the crossroads you think of as inconsequential—the decisions about donuts and burritos and M&M's—sets your compass and grounds you," he said. "When you start paying attention, you're going to find that your body has a gut feeling about virtually every decision you face, big or small. Once you begin to trust that feeling enough to act on it, this technique will be a very useful guide."

"So I'm in for a lot of donut crossroads and a lot of trial and error," I said.

"I told you this is a rudimentary guidance system. But with practice you'll get pretty good at it. Of course, once you can use the Field, all the guesswork is taken out."

"Why not just show me how to use the Field?"

"Crawl first, then walk, then run." He folded my wish list and returned it to his shirt pocket. "So, why do you think you had a headache this morning?"

"It couldn't have been anything I ate. I skipped breakfast."

"Bingo! Your body responds to what you do as well as what you *neglect* to do. When you skipped breakfast, you failed to fuel the machine. So I ask you, 'budding master of the second level,' what message was your headache delivering?"

"Eat?"

"You're a genius." Nate stood and stretched from side to side. "That's enough for now. I want you to practice listening to your body. Pay attention to its signals. When you receive one, positive or negative, ask yourself the question, 'What is my body telling me?'"

"I'll do my best," I said.

Nate sensed my lack of conviction. He let out a sigh and sat back down. "Look, just begin to pay attention. The body will interpret that small gesture as your willingness to honor the agreement you made with it at birth—to listen and respond. You'll see, in no time even the faintest signals will become clear."

"All I have to do is pay attention?"

"That's it. Here, I'll give you an example. When you were a kid, did you ever try smoking cigarettes?"

"Yeah, I was sixteen. My friend and I decided to sneak some from his mom's purse. At the time it seemed like a pretty cool thing to do."

"How did it turn out?"

"We coughed so hard our lungs ached. And my throat was scorched."

Nate smiled. "Pretty cool, huh? So, how many years did you smoke?"

"Are you kidding? I gave it up that day."

"Very smart, what about your friend?"

"He kept smoking. After a while, he could inhale with no problem. I guess his body got used to it."

"Like hell it did. Those warnings, the physical symptoms, stopped because your friend was unwilling to listen and respond." Nate put his hands up as if he were working sock puppets. "Here's the way that conversation went."

He flapped his right thumb and fingers and threw his voice up an octave.

"Inhaling smoke is cool and grown-up."

He flapped his left hand and dropped the pitch.

"Gag, burn! No, stupid, this stuff is terrible for my heart and lungs. Please stop!"

Then back up into a maniacal falsetto.

"Pipe down, will you? I'm gonna smoke whether you like it or not."

Nate laughed at himself, took a deep breath, and dropped his hands to the table.

"Pretty soon, your friend's body recognized the futility of any further warnings and stopped sending symptoms. Then he was free to inhale carbon monoxide, carcinogenic chemicals, tar, and nicotine to his heart's discontent."

"Burning and choking are powerful symptoms—kind of hard to miss. But you and I are talking about much subtler stuff," I said.

"Not really. A child's body is very vocal about its likes and dislikes. Fed the wrong food it will cry out with stomach and intestinal pain, skin rashes, ear infections, and allergies. Hard to miss, wouldn't you say? A wise parent will heed these warnings and change the child's diet. But if the symptoms are ignored—or, worse yet, suppressed with medicine—and the parent continues to feed him inappropriately, his body eventually stops yelling. The cry fades to a whimper and the behavior becomes habitual. That's when the real damage begins."

I thought about Zoë's colic. "My wife and I just had a baby girl," I said.

Something about that news gave him pause. His eyes softened and he looked at me for a long moment as if that information shed a new light on things.

"What's her name?" His voice was almost a whisper.

"Zoë," I said.

He repeated it softly. "Wonderful name. It means 'life,' you know." He gazed down at his lap, where his hands now rested, and became very still. It seemed as if something was playing in his mind. Nearly a minute passed.

"Well," he said straightening himself, "how is little Zoë?"

"As a matter of fact, she cries a lot. The doctor tells us it's probably colic."

Nate shook his head. "I suppose he told you there's nothing you can do about it."

"Is there?"

"There's always something you can do. I assume your wife…what *is* her name?"

"Merry, like Christmas."

"I assume Merry is breastfeeding."

"Uh-huh."

"Good. It's likely Merry is eating food Zoë's digestion can't handle. For the time being, she should stay away from cow's milk, wheat, onions, and garlic. And ask her to avoid cruciferous vegetables—cauliflower, cabbage, Brussels spouts, and broccoli." He reached into his back pocket and pulled out a scrap of paper, "Pick this up at the health food store."

He scribbled something down and handed it to me.

"Bifido infantis?" I guessed at the pronunciation.

"It's friendly bacteria for Zoë's bowel," he said. "Nature hates a vacuum. A deficiency of these guys isn't common in breastfed babies, but it can happen. Have Merry express some breast milk and bottle feed Zoë twice a day with a quarter teaspoon of the powder. That should do the trick."

"Thanks." As I stuffed the paper in my pocket, I realized how much I was coming to trust the old man.

"Getting back to our lesson," Nate said, "warnings unheeded will eventually fade. But one day, at about your age, those habits established in childhood begin to take a heavier toll. Energy sags, weight balloons, aches and pains multiply as the tissues and systems of the body start to fail. This new batch of symptoms, which should sound familiar to you, is a warning from the body of the growing danger."

"Jesus, you make it sound like I'm on my last legs."

"Not quite. You could ignore your symptoms and hobble along like this for another thirty years before something vital gives out."

"Oh, that's reassuring."

Nate laughed. "The good news is it's not too late to begin listening and responding."

"I don't know. I have a lot of practice ignoring my body. I'll probably miss what it's trying to tell me."

"Don't worry," he said, getting up from the table. "Your body yearns to be well. It constantly strives for harmony and balance and understands that achieving them requires collaborating with you. Your current symptoms are a reflection of the body's desire to re-establish communication. The instant you decide to participate in the healing process, it will respond by turning up the volume of its messages. I doubt you'll miss them."

He grabbed his satchel and started for the stairs. "Please invite Heather to join us for lunch."

❧

I found the girl on a stepladder in front of a bush of snap beans. She was carefully removing the long, tender pods and placing them in a straw basket that hung on her arm. As I approached, she glanced down, smiled and went back to her work.

"Nate wanted me to invite you to stay for lunch."

"Sounds good," she replied, stretching for a bean she couldn't quite reach, "I'll just be a few minutes."

I watched her in silence, unsure whether she would welcome conversation or find it distracting.

Finally, she glanced down at me. "Have you known for long?"

"Known what?"

"That you don't fit in," she said, as if it was a given.

"What do you mean?"

"You know, that you're not like everybody else—that you're living on the fringe."

This girl dresses like it's still 1968, sings for spare change, and she thinks I'm *living on the fringe?* "With all due respect," I said, "I think you're projecting."

"Really?" She stopped plucking beans and descended the ladder. "What do you do for a living?" she asked.

Her directness caught me off guard.

"Music. Songwriting. Some production—"

"A musician? Well, Mr. Sam, I hate to be the one to break the news, but that puts you pretty far from the mainstream.

"Don't get me wrong," she continued. "Being on the fringe is a *good* thing." "Fringers are the only ones with the perspective to see what's really going on. Everybody else is so caught up in the system, so heavily invested in the grind, they'll never question or even *see* how dysfunctional the status quo is."

She put her hand to her lips. "Sorry, I can get carried away." She handed me the basket. "Anyhow, you're here, which proves you're not like most people."

It was that classic form of flattery—"We're not like everyone else." But it got to me just the same.

FOURTEEN

"What's for lunch?" I called into the kitchen from the back door. Nate turned away from a cutting board piled with vegetables and pointed his knife at a broad salmon sizzling on the broiling pan. The fish, he informed us, was the gift of a friend just back from a successful trip "somewhere up north."

I hadn't eaten fish since high school. One too many deep-fried fish sticks and I didn't need to touch the stuff again. But the fresh salmon was surprisingly delicious. Again, we ate slowly and in silence, and I noticed how the ritual of paying attention amplified every flavor and texture. A modest portion completely satisfied me.

"Nate," I said, "I want you to know how much I appreciate your feeding me."

Nate nodded and finished chewing. "I would be a poor teacher and host to let you starve in the middle of your training." He gave Heather a wink.

"All right," I said, "what am I missing?"

"Indeed," Nate exclaimed, "what *are* you missing?" He placed his napkin on the table. "That's the whole point."

I must have looked perplexed. Heather glanced at Nate and rose. "I'll take care of the dishes and let you two get back to work. Then I'm going to finish in the garden."

Nate sat back and waited for her to clear the table.

"Sam," he finally said, "I feed you to help you see the difference real food can make in your life."

He studied my face. "How long have you worn eyeglasses?"

"About fifteen years."

"How did you discover that you needed them?"

"I was with my brother. He was pointing to a flyer advertising one of our gigs that was stapled to a telephone pole across the street. Well, not only was I unable to read it—I couldn't even see it."

"So, then what?"

"He marched me directly into an optometrist's office. It turned out I was pretty nearsighted."

"And what happened when you put the glasses on?"

"It was amazing. Everything came to life—it was so vivid. The world looked like an entirely different place."

"Interesting." Nate tapped his index finger on the side of his nose. "Is it fair to say that until you wore those glasses and had something to compare your uncorrected vision to, you had no idea what you were missing?"

"Exactly."

"Would you ever want to go back to that old myopic world?"

"Never."

"Sam, I feed you real food to help you 'see' what you've been missing and to encourage you to continue moving down this path you've chosen."

He straightened himself in his chair.

"Several miles east of here is a place called Hollywood."

"Yes, I've been there," I said with a laugh.

"Some of the Hollywood studios have tours of their back lots—blocks of buildings or what appear to be buildings that are used as backdrops in filmmaking."

"I've taken one of those tours." I said. "It's amazing how real everything looks."

"Realistic yes, real no. Movie folks are masters of make-believe and illusion. I suppose fantasy is harmless enough when it's used for entertainment. But that's not the case in real life."

"What are you getting at?"

He was silent for a long beat. "The world you have come to accept as real is a fantasy. It's man's fabrication, as fake as the false front of a building on a Hollywood set. That world may look real, but you can't live in it."

"Where are we living if this isn't the real world?"

"Oh, real is everywhere. But to get to it, you have to be able to look past the fake world humans have superimposed over it."

"How am I supposed to do that?"

"Over time you develop that ability. One thing's certain—to know real you have to eat real."

"What do you mean 'eat real'?"

"Real food is food in its natural form, designed by nature not man."

"You mean right off the bush or out of the ground? What about baking? What about spaghetti, or bread—you know, the staff of life?"

"Have you ever seen a spaghetti tree or a bread bush?"

"You're not too big on civilization in general, are you? People have been making bread for thousands of years."

Nate sank back in his chair and stared at the ceiling. "We're talking about the present, son, the things *you* eat. Are you familiar with the terms 'refined' and 'enriched'?"

"Of course."

"Appealing words—'refined and enriched'—and carefully chosen by marketing specialists to leave a positive impression. Read the list of ingredients on a package of bread or a box of pasta and you'll see them there. Any food lucky enough to be 'refined and enriched' must be superior to food that hasn't been, don't you think?"

He pushed the unbuttoned sleeves of his denim shirt above his elbows.

"I've got a story for you that should help make the true meaning of those two words perfectly clear." He shifted in his seat. "Ready?"

"Shoot."

෴

"One late December night in Chicago, a well-dressed man stepped out of an opera house into the blistering cold to walk the few blocks between the theater and his home. He had been careful to dress for the weather. Over his tuxedo, he wore a long woolen coat, top hat, scarf, and gloves. The man was clearly a gentleman, the picture of refinement.

"He was nearly home when a rough-looking man brandishing a gun stepped out of the shadows and forced him into an alley.

"Without hesitation, the gentleman handed his wallet to the robber who quickly removed the bills and abandoned the rest in the snow. The thief eyed the well-dressed man from top to bottom. Finally, he spoke. 'The gloves—toss 'em over.'

"The gentleman removed his gloves and gave them to the robber.

"'And the hat,' the coarse man commanded.

"The gentleman took off his hat and the robber snatched it from his hand. 'And I'll take that fine coat and scarf.'

"The gentleman was petrified with fright. Still, he was determined to avoid provoking the other man. He took off his coat and scarf and dropped them at the robber's feet.

"The bad man's eyes lit up.

"*'I've hit the jackpot!'* he thought, eyeing the fine tuxedo. He ordered the man to remove his tuxedo jacket, bow tie, dress shirt, patent leather belt, and shoes.

"Now the gentleman's exposed skin stung from the bitter cold and he began to shiver uncontrollably.

"'My new outfit wouldn't be complete without pants, now would it?' The robber sneered, unfazed by the other man's discomfort.

"The gentleman's painful, stiff fingers struggled with the pants' clasp and zipper.

"'For Christ's sake,' the robber snapped and pushed the man to the ground. He grabbed the pants at the cuffs and yanked them off.

"The robber glared at his prey. 'What the hell,' he said, 'I'll have the works.' And he ordered the man to remove his underwear and socks.

"'Thanks.' The robber kicked the garments together, scooped up the pile and backed into the shadows.

"The naked man pulled his legs to his chest in a desperate attempt to conserve body heat and listened for the fading crunch of snow under the robber's feet. But to his horror the sound stopped and then began to get louder. He struggled to stand but his numb, frostbitten feet wouldn't cooperate.

"Suddenly, the robber was standing over him, gun in one hand, the man's underwear and socks in the other.

"'*This is it,*' the gentleman thought. He pulled himself into an even tighter ball and braced for death.

"But the mugger had no intention of shooting him. He had taken what he wanted and was, in his own twisted way, feeling charitable.

"'Merry Christmas,' he snickered, throwing the underwear and socks back into the frozen man's face.

"Then he disappeared into the night."

෴

There was a long silence.

"That's all? That's the end?"

Nate lifted his water glass and took a long drink. "Yup, how'd you like it?"

"What's to like? The good guy is left naked, freezing in the cold, and the bad guy gets away with all his stuff."

"That's a fact."

"Well, where's the justice?"

"You want justice? I'm afraid you're going to have to look for that on another planet. You're sure as hell not gonna find it on this one." Nate seemed genuinely rattled. He closed his eyes and took a deep breath. "Where was I?"

"I don't know where you were headed, but we started out talking about refined and enriched food."

"Right, when food manufacturers process the grains that go into most cereal, bread and pasta, they strip out the vitamins, minerals, oil, and fiber. They call this robbery 'refining' and claim they do it to improve the food's consistency and flavor. But their true motive, you shouldn't be surprised to learn, is profit.

"Like the gentleman in our story, grain starts out fully 'clothed,' rich in nutrients. But some of those nutrients are delicate and would spoil quickly on store shelves, others would attract hungry insects."

"Well, nobody's going to buy spoiled food that's full of bugs," I said.

"Right. It's terrible for business. But the solution is simple enough. 'Refine' those nutrients out, rob the food of its valuable possessions, and there's nothing left to spoil or attract bugs."

"But then it's not worth eating."

"The insects agree. They won't touch the stuff."

"Okay, so refining isn't everything it's cracked up to be. But then they enrich it. Doesn't that fix the problem?"

"You tell me. Refining a grain removes over forty vital nutrients, enriching it involves replacing a few B-complex vitamins and iron."

I did a quick mental inventory of the food I'd been eating most of my life and could hardly think of a thing that was in its natural state. "If I gave up refined food I'd be eating air," I said.

"Hunger can be very inspirational." Nate reached into the drawer on his side of the table, pulled out a brown suede pouch and passed it to me. "But you won't need to concern yourself with eating for the next few days."

I loosened the drawstring and peered inside. Hundreds of magical algae tablets. "Now *these* are inspiring," I said. "What do you have in mind?"

He reached over and gave my hand a squeeze. "Come on. We'll finish today's lesson out back."

Thick fog rolled through the garden as Nate and I returned to the handmade table behind the house. The moment we took our seats, I had a bad feeling and buttoned up my jacket. Suddenly, I was on the verge of a full-blown anxiety attack.

I drew a fast breath through my nostrils and felt a distinct urge to run—but why?

I shot to my feet and panned the garden.

Nate sat calmly working a toothpick in his mouth.

Over my right shoulder something rustled, and I saw a strange movement sweeping through the corn, then... nothing.

Until the black and white Billy goat burst onto the path and charged directly toward us, his head lowered, ready to attack.

I looked for a cue from Nate. He was peacefully picking his teeth.

I sprang straight up onto my tree stump seat. As the goat closed in, I jumped again, onto the tabletop. When the animal was so close I could feel the energy displaced by its charge, it inexplicably veered to the right, trotted over to a giant sunflower, and began browsing as if nothing had happened.

The sight of me cowering above him proved too much for Nate. Laughing hysterically, he tipped back to get the full effect, lost his balance and tumbled off his seat. Just then, Heather dashed up the path. One look at us and she too dissolved into laughter.

"Is everybody okay?" she finally managed. "When I opened the back gate to visit George and Gracie, he rushed right in."

I jumped down from the table, thoroughly embarrassed.

"Yes, yes, we're fine," Nate chuckled as he picked himself up off the ground. "Let's tether George before he eats up all our profits."

Nate brushed himself off and righted his seat. "No harm done. In fact, George did Sam the favor of introducing him to the third level."

Heather beamed. "Well, in that case, I'm glad I could be of service." She led George away.

Nate watched them leave, then sat back to take in the clouds. He was the picture of serenity.

I cleared my throat to get his attention. "There's a *third* level?"

The question brought him back. "Yes there's a third level. It's called instinct. What sent you leaping onto that tree stump was an instinct. Fight or flight to be specific."

"How come *you* didn't budge when George came at us?"

"My instinct told me we were never in any real danger," he said. "Yours couldn't distinguish between a genuine and an imagined threat."

"Instinct," I said. "Like the swallows returning to Capistrano—that instinct?"

"Close, dear boy. Knowing without thinking—*that* instinct."

I replayed the rush of feeling I had just experienced.

"Instinct," he continued, "represents the highest form of earthly guidance. Take the swallows of Capistrano. Reducing their instinct to a migratory pattern is a gross over-simplification of third-level awareness, and that goes to the heart of the problem—man's condescending view of Earth's instinctual creatures. We fail to recognize that we're the ones who operate at a disadvantage."

"You'd think intelligence would count for something," I said.

"If our sad state has proven anything it is that we have become too smart for our own good. Look at what's happened. Paranoid and driven by self-preservation, we've mistrusted instinct and elevated our intellect. We believe we can bend nature to our will, but, ironically, we've done more to threaten our own safety than any real or imagined enemy ever could."

"What exactly *is* instinct?" I asked.

"The ability to receive nature's guidance—her instruction for us—carried on the upper frequencies of the Field of Life. Everyone's born with it. In fact, your daughter's instincts are still intact. She's a completely intuitive being, responsive to all of nature's messages." He scratched the back of his neck. "You should also know that she is acutely aware of the Field."

Those last few words gave me a chill.

"Be warned," Nate cautioned, "Zoë's instincts demand high amounts of Life Force to sustain them. With her first taste of refined and processed food, she will take her first step away from the Field and her instincts will soon vanish just as yours have."

"I won't let that happen," I insisted.

"A lost man makes a poor guide. If you want to help your daughter, first you have to help yourself—reclaim your birthright."

Nate stood and walked to the potting bench under the stairs.

"To access the third level, you have to live an authentic life, in alignment with nature's design," he said. "You'll need to relearn actions that were once automatic, one by one."

He took a few clay pots from a low shelf and began to fill them with topsoil. "Tomorrow you'll take another step toward nature's Field of Life," he said. "That step will test your resolve. I wish acquiring new habits were as easy as slipping on a pair of eyeglasses. But it's not." He pulled a seedling out of a water-filled jar and gently worked it into one of the pots. "Get to bed early," he ordered. "And call me the moment you rise. Do nothing until we have spoken. Do you understand?"

"Yes."

"Good, now go—and don't forget to take the pouch of 'pond scum' with you."

FIFTEEN

When I got home, Merry was setting out dinner—brown rice and sautéed vegetables, a holdover from her vegetarian days. I'd always considered it one of our healthiest meals, but Nate had recommended against Merry eating three of the vegetables: broccoli, onions and garlic. I decided to wait to share that news.

Zoë's squalling later that evening gave me the perfect opportunity to bring it up. Merry was willing to try anything, and she was peeved I hadn't told her *before* we ate. As penance, I spent hours with the crying baby on my shoulder, circling the couch and coffee table.

∾

It was a rough night. When my full bladder woke me at six the next morning, I'd only gotten four hours of rest. Halfway to the bathroom, I remembered Nate's instruction to talk to him before I did anything. I stood frozen in the hallway as the urge to pee intensified. Asking for permission to relieve myself seemed ridiculous, but I had made enough mistakes lately. Rather than risking another, I dashed to the kitchen phone.

It rang twice before he answered.

"Go ahead and urinate," he said, "I'll wait."

I ran to the bathroom and took care of business.

"All right," Nate began the moment I picked up the receiver. "A friend of mine owns a natural food store in your neighborhood. She makes fresh juices there. Pick up a fresh supply every morning—a couple of quarts should do."

Nate gave me the store's address and dictated a recipe for a vegetable juice concoction he called the "liver mover" that included carrots, beets, celery, parsley, and spinach. Yum. Just a few of my favorite things. "Liver mover." The name itself was poetry.

"The juice will be your breakfast, lunch, and dinner for the next few days."

"Hey, what about solid food?" I asked.

"Yes, of course. With each glass of juice take twelve green tablets."

"That's it?"

"Trust me, the tablets and fresh juice are all you need for now."

I remembered the euphoria I felt the first time I took the algae and wondered if it would have the same effect again.

"You don't want much on your agenda right now," he said. "And expect changes. I can't tell you exactly what's going to happen because it's different from person to person."

"What sort of changes are we talking about?"

"Relax, you'll probably survive. But be warned, when you stop sweeping dust under the rug and shake that rug out, dust *will* fly."

Nate's voice softened. "While you're at the store remember to get Zoë's supplement. She should be feeling much better by the time you and I meet again."

"When will that be?"

"Give me a call when you have something positive to say," he said and hung up.

SIXTEEN

Mrs. G's Natural Foods occupied a small, brick building on Wilshire Boulevard in Santa Monica, a few blocks from the ocean. A red-and-white-striped awning spanned its front, shading the neat rows of fruit and vegetable crates huddled under the store's large picture window. As I parked the car, I wondered how I managed to pass this place thousands of times without ever noticing it.

I stepped inside and a bell above the door announced my arrival.

"Good morning," someone called from the back of the store. "Let me know if you need help finding anything."

"Someone told me you make fresh juice here," I responded.

A small, middle-aged woman with shoulder-length, salt-and-pepper hair approached me. "Sure do. What do you have in mind, apple, orange, grapefruit?"

I handed her Nate's recipe.

She glanced at the page and smiled. "One Nate Special coming up. How much did you need?"

"Two quarts, please," I said.

"So, you're working with Nate."

I nodded.

"Please tell him Maggie says hello. This'll take a few minutes. Have a look around." She returned my paper and disappeared down the aisle.

The store was small—couldn't have been more than seven, maybe eight hundred square feet. It felt cozy, the complete antithesis of the cold, sterile supermarkets where Merry and I shopped. The walls here were covered with aged wood that could easily have come out of an old barn. Incandescent bulbs in green hooded fixtures hung, three to an aisle, from a stamped tin ceiling. Philodendron vines cascaded from the tops of pine grocery shelves.

The juice extractor began to whir noisily. As I wandered around the store, perusing the neatly ordered shelves, I didn't see any of the national brands I was familiar with. There were no cold breakfast cereals, no sodas, no coffee, no canned soups or vegetables. The store didn't contain a single loaf of bread.

One aisle was dedicated to teas and spices, another to herbs, oils, and condiments. I picked up a jar of olives and noticed they were grown and bottled by a small, local company.

The last aisle displayed more kinds of dried beans than I knew existed. Next to them were sacks of grain with handwritten shelf tags identifying each one: quinoa, amaranth, teff, buckwheat, millet, spelt. I counted six types of rice. Across that aisle, small bins built into the wall held a wide variety of raw nuts, seeds, and dried fruit.

I decided to look for the bifido infantis. Nate said I would find it in the refrigerated section because the live bacteria needed cold to stay in hibernation.

The refrigerators at the back of the store were stocked with raw dairy products, goat milk, yogurt, and cheese; cage-free eggs; and packages of tofu in three firmnesses. I slid open the glass door of a small free-standing refrigerator and grabbed the last bottle of bifido infantis powder.

I heard the juice extractor stop and worked my way over to the produce section that dominated the other side of the store. A hand-painted sign over the artichokes read: "All our Fruit and Vegetables are Organically Grown by Local Farmers."

"So what do you think?" Maggie asked as she handed me the juice.

"Very nice," I said. "This place feels more like a labor of love than a business."

She laughed. "That it is. That it is!"

Maggie volunteered to give me the cook's tour. Bouncing up and down the aisles as if she had springs in her shoes, she pointed to items here and there, explaining their origins and the reasons she decided to carry them. She spoke with her whole body, as if words alone were insufficient.

When we reached the register, I introduced myself and paid for the juice.

"This is your first internal cleanse," she said handing me my change.

Internal cleanse? "Is it that obvious?"

Maggie put her hand on my shoulder and gave me a gentle look.

"Just take it easy," she said. "In my experience, it's best to lay low for a day or two. Once you're over the hump you'll be fine."

When I got back in the car, I opened the juice and took a sip. It was delicious.

I can do this. A few days of magic pills and fresh juice—how bad could it be?

SEVENTEEN

The nausea struck first, followed closely by uncontrollable diarrhea. Sometime after "lunch" I found myself in the bathroom, suppressing the urge to vomit as the foulest smelling shit poured out of me.

The algae didn't deliver any of the oomph I expected. Instead, my energy drained away. I was an electronic toy with dying batteries. At some point, I must've passed out, because I woke up on the daybed in the music room that afternoon with a splitting headache, damp with sweat. The juice and those magic green pills were waging war inside me.

"Honey, I think you oughta go to the doctor," Merry said when I wandered into the kitchen. "You must have the flu or something. Do you have a fever?"

I had to tell her. "I don't think it's contagious. Nate has me drinking this juice from the health food store. Ironic, isn't it. Health food. I feel like crap. The lady at the store said something about an 'internal cleanse.'"

"Poor baby," she said, rubbing my back. "I used to have friends who did this kind of stuff. It gets worse before it gets better. But it gets better."

She stroked my forehead. "Just don't get homicidal on me, okay?"

By the second day, the diarrhea and nausea began to subside, but now I was depressed and anxious. My rotten mood soaked through every waking moment. At lunchtime, I dropped a glass of juice onto the kitchen floor and swore a blue streak. When Merry tried to help clean up the mess I lit into her.

"Leave it alone!"

"Suit yourself," she said, throwing up her hands. "We're going to stay out of your way for a while." Then she collected Zoë and left the house.

I was furious.

"That son-of-a-bitch *knew* this was going to happen," I yelled at the top of my lungs.

Another spasm gripped my insides and I raced to the bathroom.

"'You don't want much on your agenda right now' is *not* a warning," I ranted as rats, cats, and elephants stormed out of my body and into the toilet.

That evening I knew just what would make me feel better: sugar. My algae and juice "dinner" temporarily blunted the cravings, but soon they came roaring back. Somehow, I ended up in front of the open refrigerator holding a pint of Ben and Jerry's Cherry Garcia ice cream.

"Oh, no you don't," Merry said, prying it out of my hand. "If you're going to do this, you're going to do it right." She threw the carton back into the freezer and wedged herself between me and the door. "Or do I have to call that Nate person and tell him you can't handle this crazy fast?"

I laughed for the first time in days, imagining how *that* conversation might go.

"That's okay. Thanks, honey," I said, heading for the bedroom. The way things were going, the next best thing to sweets was sleep.

᪾

On day three, I awoke feeling almost human. The headache was gone, and my stomach had calmed down. After "breakfast," I noticed that my energy, though low, didn't seem to be sliding any lower.

But my mood hadn't improved at all.

I dragged myself to Maggie's store, and as she made my day's supply of juice, I described my cranky blues.

"Sounds like withdrawal," she shouted over the noise.

"Withdrawal? From food?"

"From starch and sugar," she said, turning off the machine. "You're a carbohydrate addict."

"I'm a what?"

"You've become addicted to starch and sugar. It's very common. The good news is, you're doing something about it."

She poured me a glass of fresh juice and put the remainder in a cooler behind the counter.

"Come this way," she said.

I followed her to the front of the store where she sat me down on a high stool. "Let me explain what you're going through," she said.

"The human body is a biochemical machine," she began, stepping behind the register. "For over a hundred and fifty thousand years, we ran just fine on the energy we found in vegetables, fruit, nuts, seeds, and an assortment of little crawly things. Once in a while we'd manage to take down a mastodon." She made a clubbing motion with a zucchini.

"Back then, whatever energy we didn't need immediately was stored in our bodies as fat. When food was scarce, we could tap our fat reserves and convert them into blood sugar for energy to keep us going for days or even weeks if necessary.

"But about ten thousand years ago, humans got tired of wandering around looking for food and took the production and supply of it out of nature's hands. We invented agriculture and began to grow wheat, rice, corn, potatoes, and other starches to ensure that we would never go hungry."

"What's wrong with that?"

"Starchy foods are a very concentrated, easily accessed form of energy. And I suspect they would have done us little harm if we had kept our intake to a minimum and managed to maintain an appropriate diet for ourselves."

"Nate started to tell me about this. What do you mean by an appropriate diet?"

"The one nature intended for us: vegetables, fruit, nuts, seeds, and an occasional mastodon."

"Mastodon, huh?"

"Okay, mastodon might be hard to come by. You can replace that with a small amount of animal protein if you like, but it isn't necessary."

"That's it?"

"Essentially."

"What about starch?"

"I carry a slew of whole grains because people like starchy foods, but the truth is we have no biochemical need for them."

"I don't get how you know this."

"Direct experience," she said. "You'll see for yourself if you hang in there with Nate."

"I can't imagine living without bread or pasta or rice or potatoes."

"Spoken like a true carbohydrate addict. A lifetime of eating starch and sugar has short-circuited your body's ability to manage its own fuel supply. You've essentially converted your body from a fat-burning machine to a carbohydrate-burning machine. Whenever your energy drops, instead of tapping your fat reserves for more, you're compelled to find something sweet or starchy to jack it up again. Instead of burning your fat, you end up wearing it." She pointed to my spare tire.

"All right, you win. I'm an addict. Do you think I've kicked it yet? Am I over the hump?"

"Almost." She mussed my hair. "The brain is a sensitive organ with a voracious appetite. Even the slightest fluctuation in blood sugar can make it very unhappy—that's why you've been so moody lately. The juice fast Nate put you on will do more than clean your insides, it will remind your body of its true design, teach it to use its fat for energy and break that addiction to starch and sugar. *Then* you'll be over the hump."

"Man, that sounds like one big hump," I said with half a smile.

Maggie retrieved the rest of my juice from the cooler.

"Today's supply is on me," she said, "my contribution to your future good health."

"Thank you so much." I gave her a hug.

"Do me a favor," she called out as I headed for the door. "Get yourself back to Nate as soon as you can. You don't want to fall off the wagon."

"He told me not to call until I had something positive to say."

Maggie gave me an encouraging nod. "Well, maybe you do."

EIGHTEEN

Merry was in the kitchen preparing Zoë's breast milk and bifido infantis cocktail. She glanced up.

"Feeling any better?" she asked.

"Yeah, the worst might be over. I'm sorry about yesterday."

She pulled my arms around her waist and pressed her body to mine. "I'll think of some way you can make it up to me." We kissed. "It looks like this is going to be a red- letter day for my daughter *and* my husband."

"So, it's working?"

"Your friend Nate knows what he's talking about. Last night she went down without a fuss and slept straight through. And you were out like a light."

I was happy for Zoë—and thrilled at the prospect of all of us getting some rest. But the news gave me a sinking feeling, too. If Nate was right about the baby, maybe he was right about the rest of it, as well. The "no spaghetti or bread." The endless chewing, for God's sake. The big sweep of the arm that cleared all the food I'd been eating for years right off the table. It all might be real. And it might be tough.

"That's great," I said.

Merry went back to fixing Zoë's bottle, and I decided to check on our little girl.

I found her wide awake, arms and legs in nonstop motion, transfixed by the colorful mobile revolving over her crib. As I lifted her up, she looked directly at me and smiled.

That smile was like the sun chasing off morning fog, and the roiling clouds that had clung to me for days disappeared. Nate's help had made a huge difference, and I wished I could take back all the rage I'd sent flying his direction. Those last few torturous days weren't his fault. They were payback for being unconscious for four decades.

For the next few hours, Merry and I straightened the house and took turns playing with Zoë. My energy kept rising, and after my juice and algae lunch, I felt like getting back into the world.

Merry hadn't had a moment to herself in weeks, and I knew she wanted to get back to the gym, so I volunteered to watch Zoë for the afternoon, figuring I could take her for a walk.

By the time I showered and dressed, Zoë was down for her afternoon nap, so I gently transferred her into the stroller, stocked it with everything she might need, and headed out into the day. The sun was warm; the air cool and dry. We made our way through the Spanish stuccos and modern glass boxes of the neighborhood toward the small specialty shops and restaurants along Montana Avenue that catered to well-heeled Westsiders.

I had taken this walk hundreds of times looking for inspiration, but today something was very different. I stopped the stroller and stood perfectly still. Then it struck me. All of it. Subtle aromas and tiny sounds were coming through with extraordinary clarity. Edges, textures and tonal gradations of everything under the street's canopy of palms and pines were more defined. The improvement was something like slipping on a new pair of glasses, but more dramatic, more comprehensive. The grass was greener than before, the sky bluer. I could easily judge each object's relative density by the way light played across it.

My sense of spatial perception had deepened too. Not only was I able to determine precisely where I stood in relation to every element I could see, I also knew where each element stood in relation to every other. It was as though I could see the world from multiple perspectives simultaneously.

I continued playing with my new abilities and began to entertain the remote possibility that I might be some late-blooming superhero, just come into his powers.

Would I use these powers for good or evil?

I chuckled to myself. *For good, definitely for good.*

Waiting for the walk sign at Fourteenth Street, something flashed in the corner of my eye. I turned and saw the chestnut vendor's antique cart parked a quarter of a block north at the entrance to a small shopping center. The last time I'd seen that cart I was on the verge of collapse after only a few hours without food. But here I was, three days and counting without anything solid in my stomach. My energy was steady, my mind sharper than ever, and I wasn't the least bit hungry.

I went over to say hello just the same.

Once again, the gleaming old wagon stood unmanned. But the sign on the front had been changed. It now read:

Cool Lemonade - $1.00

I figured this couldn't be the same vendor I had met at the Promenade and was about to walk on when I noticed the small, scalloped-edged card on the left side of the counter directing the reader to "Ring Bell for Service."

I rang the bell and waited. Nothing happened.

Suddenly I felt very thirsty. It was nearly an hour since we left the house, and I had remembered to pack everything but water.

I rang the bell again and peered across the counter, half expecting the man to materialize out of thin air. A double sink occupied the spot where the grill had been. To its left, a cutting board lay next to an old-fashioned, pump-handled juice extractor. Two clean glasses rested upside-down on a white terry cloth dishtowel.

I heard Zoë stir and knelt down to make sure she was all right.

"A brand new life—so much potential," a familiar voice boomed overhead.

"Jesus!" I yelled, falling back on the sidewalk.

"Actually, the name's Noah," the voice called down. "I apologize for frightening you. Sam, isn't it?"

As I pulled myself up, I looked directly at the man and was struck by how much his appearance had changed. He wore dark sunglasses, a broad-rimmed straw hat, white Bermuda shorts, and a colorful Hawaiian shirt. His posture, so formal before, was now completely relaxed. If it weren't for his distinctive voice, I wouldn't have recognized him.

Noah pulled the sunglasses to the end of his nose and studied me.

"You look thirsty," he said. "How about a nice cool glass of lemonade?"

"Sounds good," I replied. "But I'm on a vegetable juice fast and—"

"Aha!" he exclaimed. "No wonder your light is shining so much brighter."

"My light?"

"The last time we met you were a pretty dim bulb."

I cast my mind back to that moment. "Yeah, I guess I was."

"We must celebrate your illumination with some lemonade," he insisted.

"I don't know if I should."

"You rang the bell, didn't you?"

"Yes, but—"

"Wasn't your last purchase to your liking?"

"The chestnuts were great, but this is lemonade."

"Lucky for you I operate this mobile refreshment stand with a very flexible business model. Today you don't happen to need chestnuts."

"You think I need lemonade?"

He put his elbows on the countertop and rested his chin on the back of his hands. "Someone needs to learn to trust his Self."

His Self? I was too thirsty to worry about grammar. Besides, this would be a perfect opportunity to test my second-level awareness. If the lemonade was a bad choice, my body would tell me.

"All right," I said, "one lemonade, please."

Noah pushed the sunglasses to the bridge of his nose and tipped his hat.

"Yes, sir."

He reached under the counter and produced two beautiful lemons, which he carefully split in half. Then he set the halves into the extractor and pressed the juice out of each. Every movement seemed measured, every action deliberate. For this guy, making lemonade wasn't so much a task as a ritual.

"That's an awful lot of work for a glass of lemonade," I said.

"It can only work its magic when it's fresh." He poured the juice into a metal shaker, added a scoop of ice and splashed in water from a carafe.

"Now for the finishing touch." He pulled a small sack from under the counter. "This is stevia." He sprinkled a tiny spoonful of fine white powder into the cup. "This wonderful herb has all the sweetness of sugar and none of the nasty side effects."

He sealed the cup and began to shake it. His whole body got into the act, swaying to the calypso rhythm he was creating, and soon he began to sing. "If somebody wants a treat, first he has to move his feet. When somebody moves his feet, he will surely get a treat."

Noah was making a complete spectacle of himself. But oddly, none of the passersby so much as glanced at him.

The man's exuberance was infectious, and I lifted Zoë out of the stroller, cradled her in my arms and sidestepped back and forth to the joyful sound.

The rhythm stopped.

"Soup's on," Noah called, straining the cool mixture evenly into two tall glasses.

I picked one up and handed him a dollar bill.

"Here's to your health," Noah said, lifting his glass.

"And yours!" I took a sip. The drink's intense flavor, sweet and sour, exploded on my tongue.

"Wow. That is good."

"Good and good for you," he crowed.

"I have a friend who says that," I said, taking another long sip. "You'd like him."

"No doubt I would. Now finish up."

I drank some more and watched him clean the cutting board.

"Lemons have a special quality all their own," he said, wiping the board. "Every other food weighs us down, pulls our body to the ground. Eventually, it is food that drags us back into the earth. But not lemons, lemons lift us up."

"You mean up in the air?"

"That all depends on how high one is ready to go."

He plunged his towel into the sink, gave it a wring and turned his attention to the extractor. "This vegetable juice fast you are on has lightened your body's load considerably." He removed his sunglasses and peered at me. "Yes, my lemonade was exactly what you needed. Now let me have that glass."

I took the last tangy sip and handed it over.

"Noah, that friend I mentioned—his name is Nate. Do you know him?"

Noah washed the glass in the left sink's soapy water.

"And the biofield," I rushed on. "Do you know about that too?"

He dipped the glass into rinse water and held it up for examination. "Yes, I know." He pushed in a dry towel and gave it a turn. "Perhaps one day you and I will speak of it." Then he trailed off. "But not today."

He knew! Say something, anything.

"I bet you'd sell a lot more lemonade if you served it in paper cups people could take with them."

"And give up the satisfaction of cleaning this glass? Never! Besides, the visit is half the fun." He gave me a wink and began to dance again to music only he could hear.

Being with Noah felt so good, I didn't want to leave.

"Go, go," he sang, shooing me away. "It's time you were getting home."

Reluctantly, I placed Zoë in her stroller and headed back toward Montana Avenue. The walk to the corner couldn't have taken thirty seconds, but when I looked back to wave good-bye, Noah and the cart were gone.

NINETEEN

I was so preoccupied with my visit with Noah and his impossibly quick disappearance that I found myself pushing the
stroller up our front walk with no recollection of how I had
gotten us there.

Merry wasn't home and Zoë was hungry, so I pulled some
breast milk out of the freezer and warmed it up—everything
her body needed, right there, provided by nature.

We sat on the couch as she finished the bottle and went
straight to sleep in my arms. I studied her face and watched
her breathe for awhile before my own fatigue overtook me.
Settling her on my chest, I sank back on the deep cushions
and closed my eyes.

෬෨

A breeze whispered into my consciousness. Almost inaudible
at first, it gradually intensified until the sound of rushing air

became deafening. Then a high, sharp call pierced the din and my eyes flew open. A rural landscape was racing by hundreds of feet below me. Strangely, though I'm deathly afraid of heights, I was calm. I had the reassuring sensation of being held securely aloft by powerful and tangible air currents, as if I were a ship afloat on layers of invisible water.

From this altitude, the hills, bathed in late-afternoon sunlight, appeared to fold into one another, their surfaces obscured here and there by small stands of trees etching long shadows along the slopes or nestling in the darkened crevices between them.

An updraft gently lifted me through a wisp of cloud, then retreated, allowing me to coast downward again in long, lazy circles. Straightening my flight path, I rode the wind westward as the land below gradually flattened to a patchwork of green and gold fields.

Again I heard the piercing call and my eyes caught a tiny brown speck, racing across an open meadow. With a surge of adrenaline, I plunged into the suddenly receptive air. Faster and faster I dove toward the moving speck, instantly matching my trajectory to any change in its course.

The ground drew closer, the speck grew larger and I recognized my target. It was a field mouse, running for its life—running from me. With one great thrust, I propelled myself the dozen feet that remained between us and pounced on the frantic animal. It squirmed in my grasp as I pushed off the ground and was airborne again, gliding low over the meadow for a moment before an updraft sent us skyward.

I banked to the right and caught sight of my next destination. On a mountaintop east of the valley, a single pine towered over the other trees. Something or someone waited for me there; I was sure of it. Now the same invisible forces that transported me down to the meadow gathered once again to guide me through the shifting winds to that distant mountain.

The long flight took all my energy. Even so, I spent one last moment circling high above the giant tree, surveying the area the way a pilot might before landing. Satisfied that all was as it should be, I swooped down.

In the uppermost branches, a magnificent red-tailed hawk and her chick huddled together in a nest that glowed with the last rays of sunlight. As the birds looked on, I landed and carefully released the fresh kill onto the nest's floor. The hawk retrieved the gift, fed the chick and took a few bites for herself. Then she nudged the mouse my way as if to say, "You should eat too." I took a small bite of the still warm animal, then another and another. With each bite, I felt my strength returning.

The wind subsided. As I glanced west, darkness spread across the far side of the valley.

A hush came over the mountain.

The nest rocked gently in soft, cool gusts.

Cradled high in the tree, a feeling of complete contentment came over me, and I knew that this place between heaven and Earth was where I belonged.

I rested beside the hawk and her chick as the crickets, toads, and songbirds of the forest began their delicate and beautiful accompaniment to nightfall.

TWENTY

A t first light, I called Nate, eager to tell him everything
that had happened since our last meeting: the bleak start
with nausea and diarrhea, the crashing fatigue and withdrawal
symptoms, coming back to life with newly acquired "superpowers," dancing with Noah, flying in my strange dream.

When I finished, there was a long silence on the other
end of the phone.

"Come on over, and wear your sneakers," he said as he
hung up.

I arrived to find him sitting on his porch steps, loading
apples into his satchel.

"You look good," he said, passing me a piece of fruit. "I
assume you haven't had breakfast."

My mouth filled with saliva. "I haven't eaten a solid thing
in days."

"Break-fast. Now *that's* an aptly named meal. Not to be
missed, in my opinion. Well, go on, eat. You're going to need
your energy."

I sank my teeth into the crisp apple. Sweet, tangy juice swept across my tongue.

Nate stood. "Of course, if you prefer, I think there might be a donut somewhere around here."

We looked at each other and laughed. "It's amazing how little I want one right now."

"I'll tell you why," he said. "Unlike that apple you're enjoying, a donut has nothing of value to offer you. Your body has always known that. Now you do, too."

I found it odd that Nate should refer to me and my body as if they were separate entities.

"Your old, deadened sense of taste might've craved such things, but not your new, sharpened one," he continued. "Improved reception on the first level of awareness, what you call your new 'superpowers,' is a sure sign you're on the right path. And you can expect to receive more messages on the second level as well."

"Yeah, my body has been doing a lot of talking over the past few days. Yelling, really."

"The first step back to the Field can be difficult for some folks. Usually a person's discomfort is directly proportionate to the amount of garbage they're carrying."

"It felt like I was unloading a *lot* of old stuff."

"The residue of decades of indiscriminate and excessive consumption. Garbage in, garbage out."

Nate turned and strode toward the north side of the property. "Come on," he called over his shoulder, "I want to tell you a story."

He moved quickly and easily through the brush. I raced after him, tripping on exposed roots, slipping and sliding through wet leaves. About fifty yards in, he stopped at the head of a trail that led through an open field toward the Santa Monica Mountains to the east.

"Try to keep up," he called, "we've got a lot of ground to cover."

I quickened my pace.

He took off down the trail, and as he spoke, he directed the words out across the meadow as if they were intended for everything within earshot:

"Once upon a time, there was a splendid metropolis. Its buildings, parks, and residences were all beautifully designed. Its streets were wide and well maintained. Every item bought and sold in the city was well crafted and designed for permanence. For years, the metropolis thrived.

"Then one day its leaders decided that good wasn't good enough. The city needed to grow, to be bigger than all its neighbors, and to grow it needed money.

"'How will we do that?' the merchants asked. 'People only buy what they need, and everything lasts a long time.'"

Nate paused to address a bush. "'I know!' said one, the sign painter who helped people advertise their wares. 'We can craft shiny new goods and give them to our wives and children. When they show off these rare things, which will be fancy but flimsy, other people will want them. They'll have to have them!'"

"The city elders were skeptical, but they tried the man's trick. And they were astonished when the people in the town began begging for the new goods. Sooner than anyone expected, people forgot their traditional frugality and clamored for what was new, just because it was new. Soon, the townspeople and the now-much-wealthier merchants were calling permanence 'old fashioned.'

"Having the latest, most advanced possessions became the new mark of status. Even food changed, and it too was subject to fads and crazes. The new restaurants that went up all over the city sold this 'fad' food in disposable containers. New shopping districts popped up, peddling dazzling but poorly manufactured goods that required regular replacement."

Nate stopped for a moment at the end of the field where the trail turned downward into a canyon that lay between his mountain and the adjacent one.

"The economy grew and, with it, the city's coffers. The merchants praised one another for their vision, and they made the sign painter mayor of the city. No one thought beyond the magical wealth they'd created to consider the consequences of this new way of life."

He started downward.

"The citizens now spoke of themselves as 'consumers,' and the more they consumed, the more garbage they generated. Soon the growing trash pile proved too much for the city's sanitation department. Its overworked employees became sick; their trucks broke down from excessive wear and tear.

"A few concerned officials proposed a moratorium on consumption to reduce the amount of trash and give the city a chance to catch up on garbage removal. But their colleagues in city hall, giddy with prosperity, rejected the proposal."

Nate stopped. "So, what do you think happened?"

"I imagine the garbage men went on strike," I said.

"Bingo. Fed up with the abuse, they walked out."

He turned onto the final switchback. "Within days, garbage began to spill into the streets, making it impossible for anyone to get to work. Businesses failed, neighborhoods deteriorated. Soon, the once gleaming and prosperous city stood on the verge of collapse."

Moments later, we reached a narrow creek at the bottom of the canyon. Nate sprang across, surefooted as a mountain goat.

"Well," I insisted, stumbling to the other side by way of an exposed rock, "what did they do?"

"What would you do?" He reached into his satchel, produced two more apples and handed one to me.

"Well, if I were in charge, I'd go with the moratorium idea and give the garbage men a chance to get caught up. I'd convince the city elders to promote the value of things that last, you know—turn 'consumers' back into people. Then I would return to the old system that generated less garbage, so things could get back into balance."

"Aha!" He pumped his fist. "And that's exactly what *you* have been doing on this cleanse. Even under ideal conditions, human digestion is an inherently inefficient process that generates more waste than the body's elimination system can handle. Fact is, most people are literally full of shit."

"Nate, you are the *brightest* ray of sunshine this morning."

He ignored the jest.

"The juice fast was the moratorium your body needed to get rid of its trash."

"I don't mean to be difficult, but that's not really something you can do forever. People have to eat, don't they?"

"When man was connected to the Field, he ate only what nature provided. There was no factory farming, no supermarkets or restaurants enabling people to eat three hundred sixty-five days a year. Our food supply ebbed and flowed

SAM ROSE

with the seasons in natural cycles of scarcity and abundance. When food was scarce, man's body used the opportunity to cleanse itself of the waste it accumulated during times of plenty. Moratoriums were built into the system. Do you see?"

"Yes."

"Well, congratulations. You've just taken another step closer to the Field."

My skin tingled.

"Now, what do you make of the dream you had yesterday?"

With all the news I had brought him, it seemed strange that he should want to talk about something as amorphous as the dream. "I don't know. Why do you ask?"

"When a person has labored to open an oyster and has finally removed the pearl, he shouldn't waste too much time admiring the broken shell."

Great. Another riddle. "Okay, if you say so."

He frowned. "The next time you receive a message on the third level of awareness, don't be so cavalier about it."

The words sent a rush through me. "The third level? There was a message in there? Which part?"

"All of it."

"Wait—why a dream? That's kind of indirect, don't you think? And easy to misinterpret."

"Son, when you're fully conscious, you're far too distracted to receive third-level communication," he said. "Until we fix that problem, the dream was nature's only way to reach you."

He pulled a canteen from his satchel, tossed it to me and started up the path that led to the top of the next mountain. "I'll meet you at the summit," he called back. "Between now and then, see if you can find something to tell me about that pearl."

TWENTY-ONE

I started after Nate but quickly lost ground. Still, I pressed on, determined to reach the top as fast as I could. But my body had other ideas. The muscles in my thighs and calves promptly fatigued, then tightened and burned. After one particularly labored breath, I felt a stabbing pain under my right ribs and I crumpled forward, bracing both hands against my knees. My heart pounded, my lungs ached. Shit. How was I supposed to climb a mountain with just one apple for fuel?

"Pace yourself," Nate called from somewhere above, "you'll get there when you get there."

The climb was sheer torture. I felt as if I weighed a thousand pounds, and gravity seemed intent on pulling me down. To distract myself, I replayed my dream over and over, searching for the hidden message.

Maybe the flying meant something. Noah said lemons lift us up, and maybe that was a clue. No lemons in the dream, though. Maybe it was something simple like the time of day. Sunset. Sun setting on my old, unhealthy behavior. God, that was trite. Okay, the birds…The birds could be the key. Like maybe I was "free as a bird," free of the grip of mass consciousness, free to live an authentic life? It felt like I was writing a bad song—all my attempts at symbolism were so pedestrian.

I blundered along that way for another half hour, until at last I arrived at the summit, sidestepping the final stretch because my legs refused to work any other way.

Nate sat cross-legged, palms to the sky, looking like a wiry, blue-jeaned Buddha. He glanced up and patted the ground to his right.

"Better sit down before you fall over," he said.

I crashed to my knees and crawled beside him.

"Be still, catch your breath." He closed his eyes. I rolled onto my back and studied the sky for several minutes, waiting for my heart to stop banging against my ribs.

"So," he finally said without opening his eyes, "what do you think nature was telling you in your dream?"

"I've given it a lot of thought."

"And?"

"I have no idea."

Nate opened his eyes. "None at all?"

I shared the lame interpretations I came up with on the climb.

"You're trying to understand the dream intellectually," he said when I had finished. "Remember what instinct is: knowing *without* thinking. Here, close your eyes."

I closed them.

"How did you feel in the dream?"

"I don't know, free. Exhilarated."

"Was there any fear, doubt or confusion?"

"Not a bit."

"The actions you took, diving out of the sky, capturing the mouse and making your way up to the mother hawk and her chick, all seemed automatic, didn't they, as if they were informed by some innate knowledge?"

"Yeah, everything felt simple. It just made sense somehow."

"That's what life feels like when you can fully access the biofield. There's no confusion, no second-guessing, no hesitation—just knowing and acting on that knowledge."

"Must be nice."

"Yes, it is," he said. "Now open your eyes."

I opened them just in time to see two gulls drifting overhead. We watched them until they passed out of sight.

"Now," Nate said turning back to me, "your dream also contained a reminder about the way the real world works. We've touched on this, but evidently nature felt we needed to explore the subject further.

"The long flight to the mountaintop exhausted you, but your strength returned the moment you ate the field mouse."

"Yes."

"What do you suppose was responsible for that?"

"I don't know. Nutrients? Are you talking about something else?"

"The mouse possessed something that gave you strength. What was it?"

"Life Force?"

"That's right. When you ate that mouse, you took ownership of its Life Force. Your exhaustion was relieved by an infusion of living energy." Nate stretched his legs out, crossed them at the ankles and braced himself against his locked arms. "So, the message nature wanted to make sure you received was simply this: Life feeds on life. Life Force perpetuates Life Force. Is that clear?"

"Yes. Living things eat other living things, and that's what keeps life going."

"All right then, where did the mouse obtain its Life Force?"

"From the grasses and seeds of the field."

"And where did the grasses and seeds get their Life Force?"

"Didn't you say they get it from the sun?"

"Only the simplest plants are capable of making Life Force from sunlight and water. More complex plants require the additional energy they collect from the soil. Did you know that soil contains Life Force?"

"No, it always seemed pretty inert to me."

"That's a misconception. In fact, the soil contains the Life Force of everything that has ever lived on Earth."

"Everything?"

"Where did you think all that energy goes when livings things die, up in thin air? For billions of years nature invested every bit of Life Force that wasn't needed on Earth inside it. The soil was her savings account." Nate patted the ground between us.

"You say '*was* her savings account.' What happened?"

"Man began making unauthorized withdrawals."

"What do you mean?"

"We made our first withdrawal the day we stepped away from the Field, the day we decided nature's plan for the distribution of Life Force no longer suited us—the day we began to plant crops. That moment was the birth of agriculture and may well have marked the beginning of the end for us."

He sipped from his canteen.

"Of course," he continued, "for an awfully long time the development of agriculture appeared to be one of man's greatest achievements. It guaranteed a constant food supply and allowed people to specialize in areas other than hunting and gathering. Specialization led to innovation and ultimately to the industrial and technological revolutions. With each revolution, man's influence on this planet magnified."

"Right. And we got art and music and science and civilization. I can't see how that's a problem."

Nate pointed a finger at me. "Here's the problem. The population of man, and that of every species, has always been limited by the amount of food available in a given area. Folks who study this sort of thing slapped a fancy name on the phenomenon—natural population density stabilization—but it's a simple system of checks and balances developed by nature to prevent the overpopulation of any one species."

He stood up and gestured at the land around us. "In the days before agriculture, a piece of land produced just enough food to support a finite number of life-forms, humans included. Populations were determined and regulated by the food supply. But the moment we began to cultivate crops we removed the cap on human expansion. As we multiplied and required more food, we simply usurped more of the Earth's surface, plowed new fields, and planted more crops."

He began to pace, spreading his arms wider with each step. "Free of nature's protective restraints and ignorant of the consequences, we put more and more of the planet under cultivation. In the ten thousand years since the advent of agriculture, man's numbers have exploded from three million to six billion souls. At our current rate of growth, there will be nearly ten billion of us crowded onto Earth by the middle of the next century."

"Okay, so we've thrived."

He stopped pacing and looked down at me, disgusted. "Sure, we've thrived—like weeds overrunning a garden."

"That's pretty harsh."

"Harsh? Humans are just one of the millions of species sharing this planet, yet we consume close to half of its resources. We're just one species, but we've claimed vast swaths of its surface for our exclusive use, driving thousands of other species into extinction. We're just one species, but the pollution we create is poisoning the entire world. If we don't change our ways, and fast, the consequences will be harsh indeed."

"Well, you can't be suggesting that to save the biofield we all have to go back to hunting and gathering, because if that's the case, we're definitely doomed."

He sat down beside me. "I'm not suggesting that. But the truth remains, our behavior since abandoning nature's Field of Life has been reckless and dangerous."

A billowy, white cumulus cloud drifted in front of the sun, offering momentary respite from the heat. I breathed deeply and considered Nate's words. "So, are you saying that if we'd stayed connected to the Field we wouldn't have developed agriculture?" I asked.

"No, given human intelligence and creativity, agriculture was inevitable. But I believe we would have practiced it far more wisely, cognizant of our place in the natural order. Had we remained fully connected to the biofield, we would never have assumed ownership of the Earth or its resources. Instead, we would have found ways to coexist with other life-forms and channeled our talents to create sustainable ways to satisfy our needs."

"But that *is* happening. Look at the way alternative energy is taking off."

"What, man's feeble attempts to address the looming specter of climate change? Hell, those Band-Aid remedies won't fix a thing until we recognize and repair the damage we're doing to the Field of Life."

"I don't know, Nate. I can't see Congress passing laws to save a field of energy they don't even know is real."

"Then they must be made aware of how real it is."

"Oh, yeah. *That* should be easy."

"You're being facetious, but it isn't that difficult."

"Yeah, right!"

"Does it seem logical that man, given all his superior qualities, should be unable to access the same information so readily available to the groundhog, the anteater, the snail, and the worm?"

"When you put it that way—"

"There *is* no other way." Nate caught himself getting emotional. He closed his eyes and didn't move for a moment. Finally, he raised his hands to shoulder height and began sweeping them through the air like a musical conductor. "Nature is a giant symphony," he said. "All of her creations, from microbes to mammals, are members of a vast orchestra that has been playing her music with pitch-perfect precision for eons." He opened his eyes and dropped his hands. "Tone-deaf man has barged onto the stage and, in the midst of that amazing music, is banging on an out-of-tune piano."

"Okay, I get it. But I still don't understand how anything's going to change."

"Change will come when enough people gain access to the third level of awareness, because that's where the answers are. *That's* where the music's playing."

Nate's words and images were swimming in my tired brain.

"Look," he continued, "I know all of this is still very abstract to you." He thought for a second. "Can you recall the energy you felt when you first ate the blue-green algae?"

"I'll never forget it."

"What was that energy?"

"Life Force."

"And the energy you felt after our first meal together, what caused that?"

"I guess that was Life Force too."

"In your dream, it was the mouse's Life Force that gave you strength."

"Okay."

"Each time you consumed a food rich in Life Force you tapped into the energy of the Field and felt a noticeable improvement in your own physical and mental energy. Do you know why?"

I gave it some thought. "Because my own Life Force is so low?"

"Exactly! The greater the difference between your Life Force and that contained in the food you eat, the stronger the effect will be."

"That makes sense."

A gust of wind swept over the mountain as if to underscore that last point. I actually *had* experienced the feeling of taking in Life Force—which was different than just words. I got that. And I *wanted* it.

"Life Force," Nate continued when the wind subsided, "powers every cell, organ, and system inside you. Think of it like electricity flowing through a light bulb. The higher the wattage, the brighter the bulb will shine." I recalled that Noah had used the exact same terms, that business about my "shining brighter," when he saw me after the juice fast. "Can people see Life Force?" I wondered out loud.

Nate laughed. "Yes, they can. From what you tell me, you're just about ready to see it yourself."

He glanced at the sun as if it were a watch and stood up. "It's time to go, but first, a question for you: If finding nature's Field of Life requires third-level awareness, and access to the third level is granted only to those who possess a high degree of Life Force, what do you suppose your next step must be?"

I rocked into a squat and thrust myself into a standing position. "It looks like I'm gonna have to become a brighter bulb."

TWENTY-TWO

Nate started back down the trail. "And how do you plan to do that?"

Eating field mice is definitely out of the question.

"Well?" he pressed. "Where do you plan to find this Life Force you're looking for?"

The answer seemed obvious. "In food," I shouted and chased after him.

We were halfway down the mountain before Nate spoke again. He stopped where a flat-topped boulder divided the trail in two. "You're going to be making decisions about what to eat three times a day, for the rest of your life. How will you decide?"

I walked up to the fork in the path and looked one way, then the other. "Your crossroads technique: make my best guess and wait for my body's response."

"Eenie, meenie, minie, moe? Well, yes, trial and error would work. But, as you said, it's not very efficient. And it assumes you are completely ignorant of the facts."

Nate stepped in front of me and extended his arms, as if he were weighing two invisible objects. "Faced with a choice between the apple and the donut, which would you choose?"

"The apple."

"Why?"

"Because the donut tastes great for a second, and then I feel like shit. The apple actually tastes just as good, and it's real food."

"Ah, so you're going to eat real food—meaning food that hasn't been tampered with. Food as nature intended." He smiled. "And where do you plan to find that?"

"In a grocery store that carries..." In my mind's eye, I saw the sign over Maggie's produce section. "Organic and locally grown," I said.

Nate seemed pleased. "So, you looked around Maggie's place."

"Yeah. I like her. Nate, I get locally grown—that's obvious—but since we're defining things, organic is just like no chemicals sprayed on the plants, right?"

"That's part of it. Organic farmers respect nature's ways. They know that their crops, livestock, and by extension, we, depend on the Life Force contained in the soil. So they are careful to preserve it. Unfortunately, many farmers in this country view nature as an adversary. To them soil is just dirt. They drain the life out of their land and then pile on chemical fertilizers to make things grow and more chemicals to kill weeds. The crops that come up are so weak they can't survive to harvest without being doused with pesticides. The produce looks perfect in the grocery store, but it's nutritionally bankrupt and full of toxins."

I smacked my lips. "Mmmm…yummy!"

Nate grimaced. "You've just gotten rid of the poisons in your body. Let's try to keep them out, shall we?" He turned away and continued down the trail.

"But seriously," I yelled after him, "I think I get why locally grown is so important."

"Why is that?"

"Because the longer a crop is out of the ground, the less Life Force it's going to have."

"See," he called, "you're not so ignorant after all. The quicker something gets from farm to table the better. Did you know that this country's food travels an average of fifteen hundred miles to market and takes a week to get there?"

The trail widened, and I pulled up next to Nate. "There's something else I wanted to ask you about. When I was at Maggie's, I noticed she doesn't carry anything in boxes."

"Or cans," he added. "She doesn't stock them because there's not a whiff of Life Force in either one. Boxed and canned foods are designed for convenience, not health. The expiration dates on them are your first clue. How much Life Force do you think something's going to have after it's sat on a shelf for months?"

Nate shook his head. "My God, half the ingredients in those things are unpronounceable. They're not food; they're concoctions masquerading as food."

We reached the bottom of the ravine. I hobbled to the other side of the creek and glanced warily up the next hill.

"Come on," Nate said, "we'll take it slow."

I managed to get my legs in gear, and we started up. Nate began to whistle a melody that wasn't so much a song as a series of notes. Some were long and mournful; others were short chirps, almost birdlike. The tune's minor key lent it a sad quality. Listening, one would never guess that the person making this sound was climbing a steep grade. He seemed to glide upward as if walking on level ground. I, on the other hand, struggled along in fits and starts, pausing frequently to gather the energy to lurch forward a few steps before stopping again to catch my breath.

A few feet from the top, I lost my balance and grabbed hold of a tree branch to keep from falling backward. I hung on, immobilized, aching in muscles I didn't know I had.

"If it hurts, you're not moving it enough," Nate said, reaching out his hand.

I grabbed his arm, acrobat-style, and he pulled me up.

"That's a good grip. Let's see your hands."

I let him take them.

"What do you do with these?" he asked, pressing his thumbs into my palms and fingers.

"I play guitar every day, and a little piano."

"Your hands are the youngest part of you. Why do you suppose that is?"

"I don't know."

"Because you *use* them. Our next order of business is to get the rest of you into this condition." He dropped my hands and glanced at the sun. "It's time to eat."

☙

When we arrived at the house, he took a seat on a porch step and motioned for me to join him. "So, what's for lunch?" he asked.

"Nate, do I have to remind you who the teacher is?"

"It appears I need to remind *you*. It's nature, my boy. And your body is an extension of nature. Why don't you ask your body what it wants?"

"Ask my body?"

"That's right."

I shut one eye and stuck a finger in each ear.

He frowned. "The earplugs were for demonstration purposes only. You look ridiculous. I can't have you going around like that in public."

I let my arms fall to my sides, too tired to feel embarrassed.

"Keep your eyes closed if you like. The point is to focus inward."

I took a deep breath.

"Good," Nate said. "It's time to use that creative imagination of yours. Pretend you're sitting in a restaurant that offers an unlimited menu, and anything you imagine materializes instantaneously on a plate in front of you."

I opened my eyes and gave him a quizzical look.

"The restaurant's not out here. Let's go, what's on the menu?"

Seeing as I had sacrificed eating for the last few days, I decided I was entitled to something tasty and not necessarily healthy. What harm could it do? After all, this was only going to be an imaginary meal.

The first one to come to mind was a hotdog on a buttered bun, the way Howard Johnson's used to make them, with a side of fries and chocolate malt. Growing up, this was my favorite restaurant meal. It glowed in front of me, but the longer I looked at it, the more I remembered the way I felt right after Zoë was born. Kind of inert. Wasted.

I substituted a hamburger for the hotdog and a Coca-Cola for the malt. No sale. I removed the fries and exchanged a glass of water for the Coke. Still, it was no go.

Now what? It's lunchtime. What do people eat for lunch? Sandwiches. I conjured up every imaginable kind: turkey, ham and cheese, roast beef, chicken salad, tuna…

It all felt like too much.

I cleared everything off and focused on the table's clean white surface. Split pea soup and a salad had gone down well before. How about now?

Still too much.

Just soup?

Not quite.

Salad then.

Nope.

I needed to eat *something*. What the hell did my body want?

Something light. Easy to digest. No big surprises. Maybe…some fruit. Just not another apple.

I pictured a bowl of fresh berries.

Blackberries, yes! And something else, a little more substantial.

I opened my eyes. "Blackberries and goat yogurt."

"*Tres bon, Monsieur,*" Nate said with an awful French accent. He stood and draped an invisible towel over his forearm. "Excellent choice, if I do say so. Now, if *Monsieur* wouldn't mind picking zose berries. He'll find zem along za fence on za south side of za chateau."

"Thanks for nothin'," I said, getting to my feet. "Don't expect a tip."

He dropped the accent. "Lucky for you, I'm not in this for the money. Let's go." We walked through the house into the kitchen where he handed me a small metal pail. "It's the end of berry season, but there should still be enough for the two of us."

◦◦◦

We enjoyed our lunch without conversation, as Nate's old radio played soft, classical music. The meal was precisely what my body wanted—light enough for my stomach to handle after those juice-only days, but solid enough to satisfy my hunger. Like most things that seem simple and obvious in retrospect, consulting my body *before* deciding what to eat made complete sense.

We finished eating.

"You're in terrible shape for a man your age," Nate said, rising to clear the dishes. "Come to think of it, you're in terrible shape for a man of any age."

Now I was embarrassed. "Move it or lose it, huh?"

He walked the bowls into the kitchen and returned to his seat.

"Not just move it, move it the way it was designed to move. "There are no shortcuts to getting in shape. But it shouldn't take too long."

"You want me to join a gym?"

"I'm not a big fan of gyms, at least how most people use them. Hell, the way the equipment in those places isolates muscle groups, you'd need a degree in exercise physiology to avoid doing yourself more harm than good."

"I don't know, Nate. There are millions of gym rats who would disagree with you."

"The 'gym rats,' as you call them, deserve a lot of credit for making the best of a bad situation. But, the fact remains, exercising on those contraptions isn't natural."

Here we go again. "So, what *is* natural?"

"Come with me."

I followed Nate onto the front porch. He stopped just short of the steps, folded his arms on his chest and scanned the area in front of the house. "Just watch," he said.

I moved next to him and stared into the trees. "What am I looking for?"

"Shhh. Tune in to the first level of awareness and see what you pick up."

I took a deep breath and mentally put all five senses on alert. Immediately, a small bird caught my eye. It flitted from tree to tree in quick bursts and then darted out of sight. I looked toward a rustling in some dry leaves nearby and watched as one squirrel chased another around the base of a pine next to the porch. Then the two of them shot straight up the tree, unfazed by gravity, and continued the chase in the upper branches. A soft crunching sound drew my attention to the ground in front of us, and I looked down in time to see a brown lizard scurry under the steps.

"Nate—"

"Shhhhh. Keep watching."

A hummingbird hovered in midair on wings moving impossibly fast and began to make the rounds of the flowering plants that hung from the roof's beams. In the eaves, a spider was busy spinning a huge web. A bee buzzed past my ear. A butterfly floated past. Between my feet, hundreds of ants marched in single file across the porch's floorboards;

some carrying objects several times their size. Everything seemed to be in perpetual motion.

I glanced at Nate, who was focused on something in the woods. "There," he whispered.

I peered into the brush. "What?"

His eyes remained fixed straight ahead.

I looked again. Camouflaged in a thicket, a coyote stood perfectly still, transfixed by something between it and us, a rabbit. Suddenly the coyote leaped forward. The rabbit shot across the clearing. In an instant, the coyote closed in and pounced, a split second too late, as the rabbit disappeared under a fallen log.

Nate turned to me. "Well?"

"What, you want me to start chasing rabbits?"

"Don't knock it. Chasing rabbits is damn good exercise. Not so long ago, your survival would have depended on catching one."

"Thank God for progress," I said.

"Stop for too long out there and risk becoming someone's lunch," he said, drawing a finger across his throat. "Before we turned our back on the Field of Life, humans were a part of that world. We thrived on the physical activity life out there demands. We didn't need to 'go exercise.' Life kept us in shape."

"But that was then," I said. "I can't complain about not having to run from something that wants to kill me. But I can see I have to do something. The question is, what? And how much?"

"Well, let's see." Nate stroked his chin. "How many hours a day do you spend playing the guitar and the piano?"

"Two or three."

"That'll do for starters."

"Oh come on. Exercise for two or three hours a day?"

"No, not *exercise* that long. Be active. There's a big difference between the two." Nate gestured to my fingers. "Your hands are strong because you play the guitar and piano every day. You practice scales the entire time?"

"I play songs, mostly."

"Right. Practicing scales is exercise. Not much fun, as I understand it."

"No, but you have to do it if you want to be a great player."

"That's a good point. Got any plans on going out for the Olympics?"

"It's a little late for that."

"All right then. I think we can forgo the complicated workout."

"Still, being active for two or three hours a day seems excessive. Jesus. It's totally impractical. I don't know anybody who does that. Ninety percent of the population would have to quit their jobs."

"Impractical, huh?" Nate stepped in front of me, cupped his right hand over my eyes, placed his left at the base of my skull and pressed. A warm charge surged through my head, evaporating every thought.

"*This* is impractical," he said, his voice sounding as if it had arrived from the other side of a long tunnel.

Gradually, I became aware that Nate had removed his hands, but my body was so relaxed it took a moment before I could get my eyes open. My head had fallen forward and I found myself staring at my feet. Then it dawned on me that I was no longer standing on the porch. I turned around to get my bearings.

There was no porch.

There was no house, no orchard, and no garden—only scattered brush where they had all been.

Nate was gone too.

"This has to be a hallucination," I said out loud. "That, or he's hypnotized me."

"What's the lesson?" I heard an inner voice ask.

"I don't know, maybe, never cross an old Indian?"

"What's missing here?"

I scanned the area.

Everything was eerily still—as if time had stopped.

I took a deep breath. The air was crisp and fresh.

I listened for a hint of activity, but the only sound was the faint rustling of leaves.

I sharpened my focus and took another look around.

Nothing moved.

No birds flew, no bees or butterflies meandered. No squirrels or rabbits raced through the fallen leaves. I knelt down to examine the ground. No ants. Not a lizard.

"This is the world in which every other creature has followed man's lead," the voice said.

"What do you mean?" I asked.

"Your species is, without a doubt, the laziest on Earth. For the past ten thousand years, every advancement, every invention has been calculated to allow your race to become less active. To make life 'easier.' In the most 'developed' parts of your culture, automation and mechanization have rendered physical labor nearly obsolete, while more and more of you aspire to sedentary lives behind desks. It seems some of you won't be satisfied until you have found a way to avoid moving even a single muscle.

"*Out there, you can see what would happen if animals lost speed, agility, and endurance—those qualities so many of you associate only with athletes.*

"*Not one would have survived. And of course, without other creatures to support the chain of life, your species would have perished as well.*"

The silence all around felt eerie now.

"*All that survives is what you see here, rooted in the ground: the trees, brush, and long grass designed for immobility.*"

I wanted to run, but couldn't take a single step.

"*In your current form, there is no place for you here. And so, you must join the rooted creations. That shouldn't be much of an adjustment for you. After all, you have lived most of your life nearly as immobile as a plant.*"

A crippling pain gripped my feet as roots burst out of my sneakers, tangled themselves around my ankles and dove into the ground around me.

This had gone far enough!

"Nate!" I yelled. "Whatever you're doing, *stop it*!"

My knees became rigid and my hips locked. I grabbed both legs and watched in horror as they fused together into a single, inflexible stalk. I could feel the paralysis spread to my waist, across my chest and up my spine to my neck. My arms jerked skyward and froze there.

"No, no," I screamed as everything went black.

∽

"No, no what?" At the sound of Nate's voice, I went completely limp and collapsed.

"What's wrong, son?" he asked, squatting next to me.

158

I rolled over, dripping with sweat and stared at him. "Don't tell me you had nothing to do with this."

"I have no idea what you're talking about," he said. "Son, you're tired. Go home and get some rest. I'm gonna need your help tomorrow."

I struggled to my feet and took a few steps, a simple act for which I had renewed appreciation. "Okay, I'll rest for awhile, but then I'm definitely going to take a walk."

TWENTY-THREE

When I got home, Merry was on all fours in the living room, playing peek-a-boo with Zoë around the coffee table. Over the next hour, I alternately joined in and watched, but my energy faded with the daylight. By six o'clock it was all I could do to pull myself from the couch and make my way to the bedroom for a nap.

Through the closed door, I heard Merry's playful voice eliciting excited giggles from Zoë, and it sent a momentary pang of guilt through me. It would be one thing if I had to be away from my wife and daughter for work, but this *thing* I was doing with Nate was something else, and I couldn't shake the feeling that I was being negligent as a husband and father. But I was too tired to dwell on it. Within a few minutes, I fell asleep.

༄

I felt a tug on my shoulder and opened one eye to the early morning light. The air was cold. I pulled the covers back over my head and rolled over onto my stomach. Then came another, stronger tug and a male voice said something in a strange language that I somehow understood to mean, "Get up, it is time."

Wait, I know that voice.

In the background, the chatter of morning birds was set at a volume I hadn't heard since childhood, waking outdoors in my sleeping bag after an overnight in a friend's backyard.

And what's this? My fingers detected something furry underneath me. Now both hands explored the surface I lay on. It felt like some kind of pelt. I pushed up onto all fours and peered out from under the covers draped over my head.

In the dim light, I could barely make out the silhouette of a man, an Indian. He spoke again. The language wasn't anything like English, but it made sense to me all the same. "Our scouts have spotted the tusked beings returning to their spring feeding grounds. It's a half-day's walk. We must leave as the sun rises."

This is not happening. I assured myself. *This is a dream.*

I realized I was wearing some kind of animal skin, tethered at my waist. I ran my hand over the fur.

A very vivid dream.

The light had come up enough to get a better look at the man who had woken me. He too wore an animal skin. He was lean, and stood about five and a half feet tall. His straight black hair hung to his shoulders. When he stooped to drop a leather pouch next to me, I took in his face—the strong jaw, high cheekbones, and chiseled features were familiar.

This guy is a dead ringer for Nate, though much younger—twenty-five, maybe thirty.

He leaned closer. "I don't know about you, but I'm tired of eating grubs." He winked as if to confirm that he was, indeed, Nate, and that he knew *I* knew that the two of us were on some adventure together. As he watched my face, he erupted with a full-bodied laugh. Then he pushed me so hard I slid onto the cold, hard ground.

I scrambled to my feet and slapped my face hard with both hands, but succeeded only in waking more fully to my dream surroundings. There were others—men, women, and children. The scene reminded me of those dioramas of paleo-Indians at the Museum of Natural History. But everything here was alive and moving. Women, wearing what looked like burlap sacks, emerged from hide-and-brush-covered huts. A few fur-clad, wild-haired children chased after them as they made their way to a nearby creek at one end of a deep ravine in which the camp sat.

I cupped both hands over my eyes, half hoping this crazy scene would magically disappear, and noticed that the skin on my face was perfectly smooth. There was no stubble, not even peach fuzz. I ran my hands over my chest and down the flat of my stomach, then around my slim waist. My body hadn't felt like this in more than twenty years.

I got to my feet. Paleolithic Nate had joined about ten other men warming themselves around a small fire pit in the middle of the camp. As I stepped into the circle, they were discussing the coming hunt—who would go, who would stay. Paleo-Nate pointed at me, indicating that I would join him and four other men in the hunt, while the rest would stay behind to watch over the women and children. He dismissed the others and instructed our hunting party to gather supplies, specifically spears, tools we would need to process our quarry, and enough rabbit jerky, dried seeds, and water to last for two days.

Although I understood all this, I didn't have the first clue where to find any of it. So I watched the other men. Each returned to his home in the camp and gathered his weapons and tools. If he had a mate, she provided him with a sack of food and an animal bladder filled with water.

I returned to the spot where I had woken. No one waited for me there. Was I even old enough to have a mate? I found a spear next to the animal-hide pouch from Paleo-Nate. The tools inside the pouch were crude, fashioned out of bone, antler, or flint, and judging from their various shapes, were meant for cutting, gouging, hammering, and scraping.

I noticed a young girl, thirteen or fourteen years old, coming toward me with a sack in one hand and a water bladder in the other. She smiled shyly and stepped very close. As she did, I saw that I was only half a head taller than her. A woman, her mother, I figured, stood about twenty feet behind her and watched as the girl offered me the sack. I accepted it. Inside was a mixture of seeds, roots, and jerky. The jerky, the girl said, was the last of her family's supply, but her mother insisted I take it to keep up my strength for the hunt. I looked over at the woman—she was beaming at the two of us—and I gave a slight bow in her direction that I hoped conveyed my gratitude.

Then the girl took the bladder's sinew strap and placed it over my head, laid it across my shoulder, and carefully arranged it at my side. When she finished she remained very close, holding me in her eyes. As she stepped back and away, her mother uttered something I understood to mean, "May the gods be with you. Come back safe."

Our hunting party headed out as daylight caught the uppermost branches of the trees at the top of the ravine. We walked single file and followed an icy creek toward the rising sun. I was fourth in line, behind three older men and leading another boy. Paleo-Nate took up the rear. When the walls of the ravine became less steep, we climbed the rocky sides to the top. My body was full of energy. I easily navigated the uneven terrain and scaled the nearly vertical wall without losing speed.

Far to the east, the sun cleared a craggy mountain range that stood at the end of a vast plain stretching north and south as far as I could see. From the topography and endless sky, I guessed we were somewhere in the American Southwest, sometime before the shift in climate at the end of the last Ice Age turned this beautiful grassland into desert.

The lead man picked up a trail heading east, quickened his step, and led our hunting party into a waist-high spray of grass. We kept up that pace all morning, slowing only for ravines and rocky streams. Lush meadows yielded to open prairie dotted with squat shrubs and wildflowers. The north wind blew cold and humid, but my body generated plenty of heat.

As we walked, the older men filled the time telling hunting stories. They took turns sharing tales handed down from their fathers or their fathers' fathers, of expeditions when game was so plentiful, a man could close his eyes, hurl a spear in any direction, and hit something. But then the conversation turned. During their lives, the elders had watched as the once massive herds of camels, antelope, horses, mastodons, and mammoths mysteriously began to vanish. Their reliable migration, season to season, had become less predictable. Now, even the wisest men were uncertain about guiding the tribe to the right place at the right time to ensure a successful hunt.

When the sun was directly overhead, we came to the edge of a thinly wooded forest that bordered the western slope of the mountains. A scout, sent ahead earlier, returned with news that he had spotted a herd of "tusked ones" heading our way from the south. We stopped to rest, circling under a small shade tree, and each man tended to his own needs. Some ate, some rested. I was hungry, but the seeds I pulled from my pouch were tough to chew, and the measly edible parts hardly seemed worth the effort. On the other hand, the rabbit jerky was surprisingly good, and a gnarly root tasted something like jicama. I took a long drink from the animal bladder.

"Save some food and water for the journey home, just in case," Paleo-Nate said softly as he knelt in front of me. I thought I saw a hint of worry cross his face. He cleared his throat and stared into the ground as if he were collecting himself. "There is a marsh nearby," he continued in a stronger voice. "The herd will make its way there when the sun hangs low in the sky. Rest, son. Gather your strength." He cupped his hands and gently placed them on my head. Then he rose, walked across our circle and began to discuss strategy for the hunt with some of the older men.

His son?

Goose bumps swept down both my arms.

My father?

166

My mind jumped in to point out the absurdity of such a notion, but it didn't matter. A sense of joy flooded in, filling the hollow in my chest that had been there ever since my father, my other father, left us.

I watched as Nate laid out his plan of attack, and I noticed how the others responded to his steady confidence. In that moment, any lingering fear of what lay ahead was replaced with love and pride. All that mattered was that I was here with him.

I lay back, following the tree's supple branches as they swayed in the wind, and marveled at my sense of contentment. I felt safe for the first time in my life.

Someone shook me awake. "It's time to go."

I sat up and scanned the camp, which glowed in the late afternoon sun. The hunting party was busy with its preparations. Nate stood in the center of all the activity, sharpening the stone point of his spear. One man unfolded and distributed cape-sized animal hides to a few of the men, another prepared torches. The boy who woke me knelt beside the torch maker and practiced spinning a fire stick between his hands. The older man raised an unlit torch and motioned to me. As I approached, he removed a glowing ember from the fire the men had built while I slept and placed it in a small pouch. He handed the torch and pouch to me, gave another set to the boy and kept one for himself.

On my father's command, everyone grabbed their spears and capes or torches and set off, in single file, for the marsh that lay farther east. No one spoke. When we reached the marsh, Nate used hand signals to arrange us in hiding places around the shore.

About a quarter of an hour passed.

I lay under a bush, nervously blowing into the pouch to keep the hot ember alive.

The ground began to rumble, the vibrations intensifying for a full minute before I saw them—woolly mammoths, giant, elephant-like creatures with long, red, matted coats. I counted one bull, three female adults, two young males, one young female, and a couple of calves. The huge animals waded into the water, and Nate signaled us to prepare for our attack. I touched the smoldering ember to the torch, igniting it.

Nate leaped into the open, waving his cape and yelling wildly. On his cue, we all jumped up and ran at the herd, flapping our hides, waving our torches, yelping and shouting as loudly as we could.

The outburst seemed to confuse the animals for a moment. But then the females closed ranks around their young, and the bull turned and charged directly at us, scattering our hunting party in every direction. Nate ran straight across its path, waving his animal hide high over his head, and drew the beast's attention away from the rest of us.

There was a heavy splash in the water. In the commotion, a young male had run farther into the marsh and was struggling in the muddy bottom about twenty feet offshore. We dropped our hides and torches and converged on him.

Two spears flew, and one of them found its mark in the animal's neck. The mammoth trumpeted in pain. Frantic now, it flailed about and managed to dislodge itself from the mud. It lurched toward shore and the safety of the herd. But the females had already made their escape northward with the rest of their young.

Panicked now, the beast spun around to fend off the circling men. Another spear flew and lodged in the animal's right side. The mammoth reared up on its hind legs, towering over us. Quickly, I moved in and thrust my spear into its exposed underbelly. The animal staggered backward, pulling me off my feet.

Let go of the spear! Let go!

My hands released the shaft and I ran into the shallow water, managing to get out from under the giant creature just before it came crashing down.

The force of its weight thrust my spear deep into its body.

There was a loud groan and then, for a moment, only the sound of my heart pounding in my ears. A thunderous cheer went up as the rest of the men discharged their spears into the motionless animal.

Exhausted, I stumbled out of the marsh and collapsed onto dry land.

"Wahwhooo! That's my boy!" Nate's hoarse, breathless voice came from somewhere behind me.

I rolled onto my belly and pushed myself back onto my heels.

At the edge of the clearing, Nate stood, bent over, exhausted from playing decoy.

Victorious, I thrust my arms into the air, and we held each other's gaze for a moment.

But suddenly, the bull mammoth rose up behind him.

"Run!" I yelled.

Nate turned, and I screamed to see him disappear beneath a blur of fur and tusks.

TWENTY-FOUR

I sat bolt upright. The bedside clock read 5:30. I took a deep breath, and my exhale turned into a sob. My trip back in time may have been a dream, but the feelings were real enough. Losing Nate was like losing my father all over again. I had buried that pain deep inside me and carried it most of my life. Now it was raw, right on the surface.

My sobbing woke Merry.

"Honey," she said softly, "what's the matter?"

"It's nothing, just a bad dream," I said, rolling over to give her a kiss. "You go back to sleep. I need some fresh air."

"Honey," she called after me as I crawled out of bed, "I love you."

I pulled on a pair of sweat pants, a T-shirt, and sneakers and stepped into the pre-dawn chill. I didn't know where I was going, but being outside would keep me close to the Nate of the dream, I was sure of it. For the first time in years, I needed to run.

"Let's move this body," I heard myself say. "Let's open her up and see what she's got." I quickened my pace and headed north on Seventeenth Street toward San Vicente, the broad boulevard that stretched a couple of miles from Brentwood to the ocean. Its wide, grass median strip served as a popular path for local joggers.

The sky was beginning to brighten as I crossed the two east-bound lanes of the boulevard and stepped off the asphalt onto the median's soft grass, enjoying the way my joints could relax on the forgiving surface. I found the jogging path heading west and shot off. As the morning chill rushed past me, I imagined I was back on that vast, ancient plain with Paleo-Nate. I took a deep breath, veered to my left and leaped over the exposed roots of an old coral tree that stood in the center of the median.

I spread my arms and, once again, I was that child flying over the hills above my parents' home. I sprinted westward along the path to the next coral tree, detouring to jump over its roots. I felt alive, young.

And then, suddenly, I didn't.

Intense pressure was building inside my skull, and it quickly erupted in a horrendous, throbbing pain. I lurched to a stop. My head felt ready to explode. A spasm gripped my lower back, my knees buckled, and I crashed to the ground— arms and legs splayed every which way.

"Hey, man, you okay?" A young woman's face, flushed from exercise, hung above me.

"Just out of shape." It hurt to speak.

"Oh, gotcha. Well, take it slow, man." She turned and took off down the path.

I tried to sit up. But the pain in my back and head made it impossible.

You idiot, what did you just do to yourself?

I'm not sure how long I lay there under the branches of that coral tree, before the throbbing and spasms subsided enough to let me get to my feet. I limped home and got into the car before Merry could see me and make me get back in bed.

৩৩

Halfway up Nate's hill, I saw him racing toward me. He pulled my left arm onto his shoulder, wrapping his right arm firmly around my waist, and practically carried me the rest of the way to the house. He carefully lowered me onto the front step.

"What have you been doing?"

"Went jogging," I said weakly. "Guess I overdid it."

"Good guess." He grabbed an Indian blanket from the porch rail and spread it on the ground. "Let's get you on your belly."

I eased down onto the blanket and lay my right cheek onto my crossed arms. "My head is killing me," I said.

Nate pressed his thumbs gently into the center of my lower back and slowly worked them up to my neck. Then he repeated the process, this time stopping in a few places to push his thumbs into my spine.

"This hurts, doesn't it?" He pressed into one especially tender spot.

"Hurts like hell."

"Uh-huh, thought so. Roll over on your back."

I did so, with great effort. "What is it, what'd you find?"

"Sit up," he said, helping me into a seated position. "Clasp your hands behind your neck and let your chin drop to your chest. Now bend your knees and allow them to fall open."

I did as he said.

He knelt behind me and threaded his arms under and through mine, lacing his fingers together over my hands. I felt his knees press into my lower back. "Just relax and collapse forward," he said.

I became a rag doll, dead weight in his arms.

"Good." He drew me toward him, arching me backward. Then, in a series of rhythmic motions, he rocked me against his knees, working them all the way up my spine. There were several loud cracks and pops. "Got it!"

The pounding in my head vanished.

"Now," he said, lowering me onto the blanket, "on your stomach."

I rolled over, slowly.

Again, he ran his thumbs up and down, finally pressing them into the spot that was so tender moments before. "How's that now?"

"Much better."

"That was a bone-headed stunt you pulled today."

"What stunt? I went jogging. Jogging's natural, isn't it?"

Nate made a hissing sound. "Yes, jogging is natural, but asphalt isn't."

I looked at him blankly.

"I know it isn't possible to avoid sidewalks and roads altogether, but stay off them as much as you can—especially when jogging. Concrete's meant for cars, trucks and buses—not humans. Think of it this way: Your body's chassis, hinges, and shock absorbers take a terrible pounding when you subject them to concrete and asphalt." He released his thumbs' pressure. "But at the moment, your body's in no condition to be running on *any* surface."

He ran his hand down the center of my back. "The nerves in here are protected by your spinal bones. Those bones rely on the support of muscles to keep them in alignment. Your muscles are weak and failed under the pressure your little jaunt put on them. That failure triggered a subluxation, or misalignment, between these two vertebrae." He pressed his palms into the middle of my spine and a tingling sensation shot up and down my body. "That subluxation put pressure on a nerve, and that caused your headache."

"I'm amazed at how you fixed it. You've got a magic touch, Nate."

He worked his fists into my lower back—he wasn't done. "Hmmm, still pretty tight, yet. When those vertebrae shifted, the muscles on either side went into spasm to keep you from permanently crippling yourself. Let's see if we can get them to unlock."

For several minutes, he worked his hands into my back muscles as if he was kneading bread dough. Finally, he stopped. "Wait here," he said, starting up the porch steps. "There's something I've been meaning to talk to you about and this seems like as good a time as any."

TWENTY-FIVE

"Come, join me," Nate said, planting himself on the porch's top step. "You should be able to get up on your own."

To my amazement, I was. I smiled sheepishly.

"That's all right. Now sit." He patted the floorboard to his right.

The deep massage left me a little light-headed, but I needed to tell him about the dream. I didn't know what it meant that I had found him and lost him in that short space of time, but it changed the way I saw him now. Changed something deeper too.

"Nate," I started.

He was holding something in his hand—his father's notebook. As I lowered myself onto the step, he opened the book's leather cover and carefully began thumbing through it. The dream could wait.

I craned my neck to get a better view but could only catch the chapter headings, all handwritten in black ink: *The Field of Life...How it Works...Real Food and the Importance of Conscious Eating...The Three Levels of Awareness...Cleansing the Internal Body...Activity vs. Inactivity.* By the time he stopped, he had paged through about three-quarters of the book. We'd covered a lot of ground.

He looked worried. "In our time together, you've learned some important lessons. But I can see that as you put this knowledge into action, you're in danger of doing real harm to your body."

His tone made me nervous. "Believe me, I won't be doing *that* again. I've learned my lesson. Next time I'll just take it easier."

Nate shook his head. "It's not that simple. I applaud the effort you made today. But your actions reflect an ignorance of your essential nature that cannot stand if you want to successfully complete this work. Our lessons have covered a wide range of topics—some tangible, some intangible. I'm happy to see that you've kept an open mind. But your next lesson is considerably more esoteric than the others, and you may not be ready to accept it."

I interlaced my fingers, raised my arms over my head and twisted, pain-free from side to side. "Oh, I think I'm ready. What have you got in mind?"

He smiled. "Let's see what my father has to say." He turned to the next page of the old notebook. The chapter heading read:

THE BODY AND THE SELF—THE DUALITY OF MAN

"Within each of us," he began, "there live two distinct entities. One of these is the physical body. It is a marvel of design, capable, if cared for properly, of transporting its occupant for well over a hundred years."

"Its occupant?"

"Shhh, just listen," he cocked his head toward me, "with your *heart* as much as with your ears." He looked back to the book. "That occupant," he continued, "is the other entity, which I have labeled the Self. The Self is our essence—ageless, timeless, and immortal. My people call this essence 'Spirit.' Yours may call it the 'Soul.'"

"Why?" I interrupted again.

"Why... what?"

"This 'entity' already has two names. Why would your father give it a third?"

Nate chuckled. "When I was his student, I asked him the very same question. He told me that people have a tendency to think of the Spirit or Soul as a disembodied component of themselves, inaccessible until they depart this Earth."

"That sounds about right."

"But it's not. The Spirit or Soul is very much alive in every one of us and can be accessed at will. He relabeled this entity the Self to emphasize that."

Nate turned his attention back to the notebook. "The Self," he read, "is an extension of universal intelligence and, as such, is privy to universal knowledge. It is the intuitive part of us, the part that responds to art, the part that creates music, the part that is moved by a beautiful sunset."

Nate laid his hand on the open page. "Are you following this?"

I liked the ideas, but found it difficult to accept something so unknowable on blind faith. "I guess so," I said.

Nate detected my skepticism. "Are you a betting man?" he asked.

"Why?"

"What do you think the odds are of being born 'you'?"

"What do you mean?"

"If your existence, your chance at life, was completely dependent on the random collision of just one egg and one sperm, given the infinite possible combinations of eggs and sperm over the course of human history, what do you think the odds are that you should ever be born?"

"They're beyond minute."

"Would you bet on it?"

We both laughed.

"Now, what if that part of yourself that you recognize as 'you' already exists and needs only to pair itself with a physical body to experience life on Earth? Do you think the odds of being born 'you' improve any?"

"If I already exist and all I'm doing is looking for a body to be born into, then, yeah, I guess the odds would improve."

I could tell he wasn't completely satisfied with that response.

He sat quietly for a moment.

"For now," he said, "think of the Self as the constant, purest expression of you—your unique consciousness, untouched by circumstance and time."

"I think I know what you're talking about. Deep inside I do feel exactly the same today as when I was a kid."

Nate seemed relieved. "Yes, that's it—the part that stays exactly the same." He turned back to the book and continued reading.

"As young children, we are acutely aware of the Self because we have just come from a place of pure energy. A child feels immortal and cannot fathom the concept of death, because for the child, who has just emerged from the realm of eternal energy, there is no death. Children's fascination with ghosts and goblins is a reflection of their struggle with the notion of mortality. However, eventually the Self must accept that on Earth, it inhabits a mortal body, which will eventually succumb to the forces that act upon it."

Nate closed the notebook. "A lot of folks never come to terms with their body's mortality. They chase immortality with prescription drugs, plastic surgery, and hormone replacement in a vain and desperate attempt to recapture their youth and forestall the inevitable."

"It's a shame we can't live forever," I said.

"The Self *is* forever—ageless and timeless. It exists before the body's birth and beyond its death. On some level, even the least enlightened of us has an inkling of our essential immortality. And that's the reason why people can be so cavalier about their health, why they treat their bodies with such disrespect, why they behave so irresponsibly. After all, the body is disposable. It is merely temporary housing, rented—not owned."

"That's a pretty ungrateful attitude. How do we get so screwed up?"

"Think about it. You know how."

"It must have something to do with our disconnection from nature's Field of Life."

"Brilliant boy! Yes, of course."

Nate reopened the notebook and continued reading: "At birth, there is total integration between the physical and the nonphysical. The Self retains strong ties to the universal energy from which it has just emerged and also has formed a strong connection to the body, its new home."

He looked over at me. "Okay so far?"

"Go on."

"The Self is pure energy," he read. "It vibrates at the same high frequency as the universal mind and is privy to all its wisdom. On Earth, the conduit for that wisdom is the Field."

"So, the Self is the part of us that communicates with the Field?" I asked.

"All our senses communicate with the Field to some degree. Only the Self is able to communicate on its very highest frequencies. However, the messages carried on those frequencies are subtle and can't compete with the incessant noise and misinformation associated with the world we've created. When that delicate signal is lost in the din, the Self becomes disconnected from its guidance system. Without that guidance, the Self quickly forgets about its responsibility to take care of the body and can become very destructive."

I didn't know what to think. I wanted to believe that some part of me would go on after my physical death, but I was still too skeptical to make that huge leap of faith. "What else does your father say?" I asked, hoping for a phrase or image that would tip the balance.

He ran his finger down the page to locate his place and continued to read. "When we are born, the Self, by virtue of its recent proximity to universal knowledge, recognizes the disparity between its own high vibration and the lower vibration of the human body, which operates at the frequency of solid objects. To make the most of its precious time on Earth, the Self understands that it must keep the body's vibration as high as possible for as long as possible. The higher the body's vibration, the more resistant it is to degeneration and disease. But the disconnected Self quickly forgets about its reliance on the body and its obligation to care for it in accordance with nature's laws. Ignorant of those laws, the Self careens through life, recklessly, with total disregard for the body's requirements and limitations."

"I see how the Self can get disconnected from universal wisdom," I said, "but the body is our home. We live there. You can't actually get disconnected from it."

Nate looked at me sharply. "The Earth is man's home, isn't it? We live here, don't we? Yet we've managed to become so disconnected that we're on the verge of destroying it. What's the difference?"

His tone set me back.

He took a deep breath and held it. After a moment, he pushed the air out of his lungs, his shoulders relaxed, and his facial expression softened. "The answer is ignorance; the same ignorance that allows the Self to abuse the body allows man to abuse this planet."

He looked over at me and scratched his chin.

"You demonstrated that ignorance this morning when you assumed you could take this out-of-shape, forty-one–year-old body and treat it as if it were still teenaged."

I felt a twinge of embarrassment. But then I remembered that I had been a teenager in my dream. It was the dream that inspired me to take that run.

"Nate, is the Self the part of me that dreams?"

The question seemed to catch him by surprise. He stared at me for a moment and then said, "You had a dream last night, didn't you?"

"Yes, I did."

"And in your dream, you and I were on a great adventure in another time and place."

I was stunned. "Yes, but how could you know that?"

Nate seemed elated. "I know because I had the same dream."

I sat there unable to speak. Finally, I blurted out, "In my dream you were my father."

"In mine, you were my son," he beamed.

He proceeded to describe his entire dream. It was like mine in every detail, except that it unfolded from his perspective.

I couldn't believe what I was hearing. "This is not possible. It's not possible for two people to have the same dream at the same time."

Nate seemed to be trying to control his emotions. "Co-dreaming is very special, very rare—but obviously not impossible. Last night our Selves took a journey together, beyond the boundaries of time and space, to relive an experience they shared long ago."

I swallowed hard. "But, why?"

"I don't know. Maybe to reinforce this work we're doing—to compel us to finish what we've started together. Maybe the dream was meant to underscore the importance of your current lesson about living an active life." He thought for a second and then added, "Maybe we were given this gift to show us that we share a bond greater than that of teacher and student." He put his hand on my shoulder and gave me a warm smile. "I'm not sure why it happened, but my heart is glad it did."

TWENTY-SIX

M oments later, we stood in the kitchen, and Nate poured a tall glass of water from a ceramic pitcher. "Here, drink this," he said, handing it to me. "That rubdown released a lot of lactic and carbonic acid into your system. Be sure to have plenty of water today."

"Yes, sir." A father's care—it felt good. I downed it in thirsty gulps.

Nate took the empty glass and set it in the sink. "Heather and I are starting a project, and we've decided to enlist your help," he said, heading for the kitchen door.

I followed him down the back stairs, past the giant sunflowers, and into the garden. We stopped at a rough rock wall that stood about three feet high and stretched from the corner of the house to a fence at the end of the property. Nate surveyed the area as if he were measuring it with his eyes.

"She wants to grow orchids, says she can sell them for a good price and raise money for college."

"That's a great idea," I said.

"And she's convinced me that it's time I moved my potting table out from under the back stairs into a proper glass house."

"You're building a greenhouse?"

"That's the plan."

I stared at the rock wall. "Here?"

"Yup, this spot gets the best sun." He pointed diagonally across the wall. "East-west orientation, southern exposure."

"But the wall—"

"Gotta be moved. Ten yards that way ought to do it," he said, pointing forward. "Then, of course we'll need to clear the brush and level the land."

"Why do I have the feeling that by 'we' you mean me?"

"Here, hold this and step back a couple of feet," he said, handing me one end of a tape measure. "According to her plans, the glass house will start just about where you are, and it'll be twenty-four feet long." Nate walked the tape out that distance. "There's only about another six feet of wall from here, so I figure we might as well move the whole thing."

"Might as well." I stared at the hundreds of rocks, some as big as my chest.

"Don't worry. I'll help you with the heavy ones." He returned and patted me on the back. "Let's go into the house. I'll make us some tea and we can go over the plans."

A sound on the other side of the wall caught Nate's attention. He cocked his head in that direction and listened intently.

"Damn it. They're back."

"Who's back?" I glanced over the wall, but I couldn't spot anything out of the ordinary. By the time I turned around again, Nate was flying up the back stairs, two at a time.

"Come on," he called back in a loud whisper.

I scrambled into the house and found him in the dining room, rolling up what appeared to be the plans to the greenhouse. He slipped them into a long cardboard tube and handed it to me.

"Take these plans to Heather. She should be at the farmer's market in Santa Monica today." Through the dining room window, we could see two large men making their way across the clearing to the house. "Tell her I'm going to need a ride home from the police station."

"Police? What the hell's going on?"

He turned away from the window and guided me by the shoulders toward the kitchen. "Oh, I got in trouble a few years back, disabled the tail rotors on a couple of county-owned helicopters. I'll tell you about it sometime."

The men stepped onto the front porch and one of them bellowed, "Federal agents. Nate, you home?"

I grabbed Nate's arm. "Federal *agents*?"

"Yeah, they show up now and then," he whispered. "That stunt put me on their shit list."

"No kidding! It sounds incredibly dumb—and dangerous."

Nate opened the back door and pushed me outside. "I'll explain later. Get behind the wall until we're gone. Then take those plans to Heather and tell her what I said."

There was a loud knocking on the front door.

"Go!" he said as I ran. He shut the door behind me and locked it. "I'm comin'," he barked, "hold your horses."

I raced down the stairs and crouched behind the wall. My chest ached, and my throat was tight.

So this is what happens when you get involved with someone from a blind ad in the paper. You wind up in an anti-government cult with a leader wanted by the feds for some kind of sabotage.

I heard the clamor of hard-sole shoes on the wooden porch and peeked over the wall. The agents had handcuffed Nate and were leading him across the clearing, onto the gravel path, and down into the canyon.

TWENTY-SEVEN

The Santa Monica Farmers' Market sprawled along Arizona Avenue between Second and Forth streets every Wednesday and Saturday. I'd never gone in, but I had unwittingly strayed into the area a few times and gotten caught in the heavy traffic around the blocked-off roads. After that, I'd always made it a point to steer clear. Today it was the usual madhouse, but miraculously, I found a parking spot on Fourth and waded into the sea of shoppers crowding the marketplace.

The event attracted all kinds of people: couples with babies strapped to their chests, groups of foreign tourists, young skinny hipsters, old hippies, salt-of-the-earth types, and women with expensive hair who looked as if they had limos waiting.

I navigated my way through the dense crowd, checking every booth for Heather. Some of the stands were elaborate, sprawling affairs with finished wooden countertops resting under massive, colorful canopies. But most were modest carts, fitted with trailer hitches or simple tables spread under small nylon gazebos or beach umbrellas.

I had never seen such a wide variety of fresh produce in one place before. It appeared as if every edible vegetable, fruit, herb, nut, and seed was for sale. And all of it had been grown nearby. One vendor offered only potatoes—more kinds than I knew existed: German Butterball, French Fingerling, Large Purple, Russian Banana Fingering, yellow, purple and red heirloom mix, and inch-long Pee-Wees.

Under a large tent in the center of the market, several folding tables lined with metal chairs served as a makeshift restaurant where shoppers could relax and enjoy gourmet tamales, roasted corn, salads, baked potatoes, falafel wraps, organic lemonade, and coffee.

With all the tumult that morning, I hadn't had a chance to eat, and my head was starting to feel hollow. This was no time for a blood sugar crash, so I ordered a roasted ear of corn and watched the vendor skillfully pull back the husk and tie it into a handle. He glazed the ear with butter, sprinkled on a little sea salt and handed it to me with a napkin. I gave him a couple of bucks and took a bite.

"That's delicious," I said. "Say, do you happen to know a vendor named Heather? Young girl, long, blond hair?"

"The hippie wannabe with the guitar?"

I laughed. "Yeah, that's the one."

He pointed west. "Her stand is on the other side of the Tehachapi apples."

෨

I found Heather sitting in a lawn chair, surrounded by a modest, U-shaped stand built from old, wooden fruit and vegetable crates, which rose progressively from the stand's open front to its closed back. The top crates were turned bottoms up to form a counter where she'd displayed vegetables and fruit from Nate's garden and orchard in simple, woven straw baskets. A blue and green tie-dyed sheet, stretched across an aluminum frame, provided shade.

She seemed pleased but not surprised to see me. "Hey, how's it going?"

"Not so good." I handed her the cardboard tube. "Nate asked me to give you this." I lowered my voice. "A couple of federal agents showed up at the house and hauled him off."

Her smile vanished. "Shit!" She pushed all ten fingers into her hair. "Fucking FBI!"

"What does the FBI want with Nate?"

She cupped her hand around my ear and whispered, "Eco-terrorism is a federal offense. Did he tell you about the helicopters?"

"He mentioned them. What happened?"

Heather set the cardboard tube on the ground and retrieved a metal folding chair from the back of the stand. She set it up next to hers, and we both sat down. "Do you remember the Mediterranean fruit fly scare we had a few years ago?" she asked.

"Yeah, it was all over the news. The authorities found two Med-flies somewhere in the valley and were worried the little buggers were going to bring down the entire Southern California fruit industry."

"So they sprayed Malathion over fourteen hundred square miles of densely populated land."

"Right. I remember thinking that seemed like a bit of an overreaction."

"Do you know what Malathion is?"

"Some kind of bug spray."

"It's a nerve toxin that interrupts communication between nerves and muscles. Exposure to it causes paralysis and death."

"The bug's death, I assume."

Heather arched an eyebrow. "Yeah, the bug and God knows how many other living things. When they spread that poison over the L.A. Basin and the Valley, do you think they even thought about the harm they were doing?"

"I never really—"

"Anyone who believes that pesticides like that won't eventually hurt other life-forms, including us, is deluding themselves."

I was struck by the gravity of her tone. "Yes," I said, "there *was* strong backlash to the idea of spraying. But that went nowhere. I remember hearing quotes from medical experts saying that the greatest threat to the public was unnecessary anxiety."

Heather let out a loud hoot and shook her head. "That must have been what sent him over the top." She smiled. "I'm sure you've noticed—Nate doesn't suffer fools."

"You can say that again."

"Well, he couldn't just sit still and do nothing. The night before they planned to do the spraying, he took apart the tail rotors of two of the county-owned helicopters they were going to use."

"Jesus, he could have killed somebody."

"Evidently, the tail rotor keeps a helicopter from spinning around like a top. According to Nate, no pilot in his right mind would ever attempt to fly without one, and you'd assume he'd notice the rotors were missing. Nate didn't try to hide what he'd done."

"So, what happened?"

"He got caught. So now the feds think he's somehow involved with every act of sabotage or destruction committed in support of the environment."

I must have given her a quizzical look, because she quickly added, "He's not. That experience taught him that you can't change the system by breaking the law. Anyhow, whenever they've got an unsolved case, they drag him in for questioning."

I fingered a leaf of kale on the table in front of me. All those times I'd seen Nate consciously stopping when he began to get worked up about something—I guess now I knew why. I could feel myself unclenching for the first time since I left Topanga. "Eco-terrorist," I said, "That's a pretty ironic label, especially for Nate."

"It's crazy, right? The people destroying the environment are painted as the good guys and the ones trying to save it are 'terrorists.'"

A young couple approached the stand. Heather lowered her voice. "They'll let him go in a couple of hours. I'll pick him up after the market closes."

As she helped the two shoppers, I noticed how enthusiastically she shared what Nate had grown. She could've sold me anything right then. As her voice went on, I became aware of a soft pulsation of light and pressure around me. When I looked up, all my senses had become heightened, just as they were a few days before on my walk with Zoë. But this time I could feel something coming through on another level, beyond my five senses. I focused all my attention into that place. It was coming from the baskets on Heather's stand.

I moved toward them and ran my hands over each one. The beans, peas, peppers, and corn all seemed to radiate faint energy in waves that tingled against my palms. Their colors seemed to brighten and dim, to varying degrees, in the same slow rhythm. I wondered if something was wrong with me, but I felt fine—great, even.

A hand came to rest on my shoulder. "Amazing, isn't it?" Heather said softly.

"Yes, what is it?"

She unleashed a laugh. Poof! The sensation was gone. "Come on," I insisted. "Tell me."

She leaned close and whispered, "Life Force."

TWENTY-EIGHT

"It comes and goes," Heather said, picking up the cardboard tube that held the plans for the greenhouse.

"What? Life Force?"

"No, the ability to see it—especially at first. You're not through with your training, are you?"

"No, I don't think so." I sat back down feeling slightly overwhelmed.

"Well, by the time you're finished, you'll be able to see it whenever you want." She slid into her chair with the tube across her lap and gave me a long look. "What is it?"

"What?"

"Something's bothering you."

I shrugged. "Don't get me wrong, I'm grateful for everything Nate is teaching me… "

"But?"

"It's…I'm getting attached to the old guy and I realized this morning that I don't know anything about him. That was kind of a shocker, the feds showing up."

She stood and set the cardboard tube against the corner of the stand. "Wait here," she said and disappeared into the crowd.

Alone in the booth, I became aware again of the subtly pulsing glow of Life Force coming from the produce in the baskets around me. I let out a sigh of relief. Staying on track with food was going to be a lot easier with the emergence of this handy talent.

Minutes later, Heather returned with a tall, pleasant-looking guy about her age. His thick, brown hair looked as if it had been combed with a rake, and his T-shirt and cotton pants appeared to have been pulled from the bottom of a laundry pile. "Sam, this is my friend Ethan. He'll watch the stand for awhile so you and I can take a walk."

As I passed Ethan on my way out, I caught the scent of patchouli oil, that trace of my idealistic past.

Heather took my arm.

"Wouldn't it be something," I said, "if everybody could see Life Force and went for what's most alive?"

"That's the plan," she said and pulled me into the flow of shoppers. "Let's go over to the park, and I'll tell you what I know about Nate."

༄

We walked a few minutes in contented silence until we reached Ocean Park, a long, narrow strip of green at the top of the Palisades cliffs on the edge of Santa Monica.

"First, a little history," she said, as we stepped onto the dirt path that snakes along the cliffs at the edge of the park. "Nate is a descendant of the Esselen Indians who lived in northern California in the mid-seventeen hundreds when the Spanish started building missions up and down the coast. A priest converted the tribe to Catholicism and used them to build the mission in Carmel. In fact, Nate's great, great grandfather was born in that mission in the early eighteen hundreds and worked in the fields there when he was boy. When the diseases the Spanish brought with them nearly wiped out the Indian population, his family escaped into the surrounding hills and eventually headed south.

"For three generations they lived and worked as migrant field hands on the Malibu, Sequit, and Topanga ranchos that were being established by Spanish land grants. Eventually, Nate's father married a young woman with mixed Indian and Spanish blood. She gave birth to Nate on a citrus farm in the San Fernando Valley."

"He told you all this?"

"He's got no kids to pass this on to. We're it. I'm sure he'll get around to sharing his history with you. I'm just telling you now because you obviously need to know."

We waited at the busy intersection that bisected the park at the top of the California Incline, a steep grade that brings traffic up from Pacific Coast Highway. When the light changed, we crossed the wide street and continued along the path as it wound farther north between rows of towering royal palms. Heather didn't speak again until we put enough distance between us and the intersection for the sound of cars and trucks to fade completely.

"His family stayed on the farm until Nate was ten, and he has vivid memories of picking oranges and lemons in the groves. But his father wanted more for his family than a field hand's salary could provide. He moved them to Los Angeles and found a job in a steel mill. Pretty soon he became the mill's foreman.

"The world was changing, and he knew that the key to his son's future was a good education. So when Nate graduated high school, his father took on extra shifts to put him through college."

"Nate went to college?"

Heather stopped, put her hands on her hips and gave me a hard look. "Yes, he went to college, and then he went on to get an advanced degree in aeronautics. The man's brilliant if you haven't noticed."

"I didn't mean to sound prejudiced. It's just hard to square my impression of him with what you're telling me. He seems so—I don't know—earthy."

She took my arm again. "I know what you mean. But he wasn't always that way. During World War II, Howard Hughes was contracted by the government to design—what did Nate call it?—a heavy transport flying boat. He hired Nate to help him build it."

"Are you talking about the Spruce Goose?"

"That's right. The Spruce Goose was the nickname the press gave it. Hughes hated that. He called it the Hercules. Anyway, it took Hughes five years to finish it, and by then the war was over."

"Wow, the Spruce Goose is legendary!"

Heather steered me to a wooden bench that faced the ocean. "*You* may be impressed, but evidently, it was a major disappointment to everyone involved," she said as we sat down. "They flew the prototype once and never built another. But Nate kept working with the company. A few years later, he met a girl named Anna who worked as a secretary in the electronics division." Heather's voice turned somber. "They fell in love and got married."

"You're making it sound like that's not a good thing."

"She was white, Irish Catholic, and nearly ten years younger than him. Her family disowned her. But they were so in love they knew they could make the marriage work. Nate talks sometimes about her beautiful smile." Heather's voice broke and she paused before speaking again. "They bought a house with a little yard in Culver City and decided to start a family. They just wanted to be happy, that's all."

"So, I take it that didn't go too well."

"Their lily-white neighbors rejected them—froze them out. Anna kept trying to make contact, but no one would even look her in the eye. Without her family, she didn't have anyone but Nate. First, she was mad at the world, but before too long her spark went out. It goes out of Nate, too, when he talks about it."

Heather looked away, telling the story, now, to the sky. "Anna stopped taking care of herself. This was nineteen forty-eight, and Nate said fast-food restaurants were starting to pop up everywhere. Anna loved them. For the first time in her life, she started overeating.

"They were both so happy when she got pregnant a year later. But she was seriously overweight by then, and when she developed diabetes, she couldn't get it under control. Her blood pressure shot up while she was in labor, and she didn't make it through childbirth." She took a long pause. "The baby didn't either."

"Oh my God," I said. That's why Nate had been so tender when I told him about Zoë and why he'd seemed so touched by our shared dream.

"So, like I said, we're it—you, me and everyone else he's helped over the years. We're his legacy."

Now I was choking up. I couldn't imagine how I'd go on if I lost Merry and Zoë. Heather stood and collected herself. "Come on, we've got to get back. I'll tell you the rest of the story on the way."

She took my arm again, but this time, it seemed, to comfort herself. We walked slowly under the rustling fronds of the palms.

Heather took a deep breath. "Nate was devastated. I don't think he wanted to live. All he could do was drink. He lost his job, his house. He had nothing." She began to cry.

I put my arm around her shoulder. "Hey, everything turned out all right."

She dried her eyes on the sleeve of her blouse. "Yes, thanks to his father."

"What happened?"

"By then he was a rich man. He had become part owner of the steel mill and made a fortune when the government poured money into this area to build factories and military bases to support the war. He took Nate in, dried him out, and cared for him until he could get back on his feet."

Traffic at the busy intersection at the top of the incline interrupted the story. "What happened after that?" I asked when we'd moved past.

"The experience changed them both. His father sold his share of the business, moved to Carmel Valley, and made the discoveries that ended up in that notebook."

"And Nate?"

"Hughes rehired him. He worked there until he had saved enough money to buy the land at the top of Topanga."

"How long ago was that?"

"Nineteen sixty, I think."

"Jesus, he's been living alone on that mountain for thirty years."

"Yeah, well…he tried the American dream, and he lost everything that mattered to him. He was done trying to fit in, done trying to be like everybody else."

"If I didn't know him, I'd say Nate was running away from life. But it's not like that. He embraces life, all life, so passionately. I think he went up on that mountain to find something to believe in."

Heather squeezed my hand. "Lucky for us, he did."

A few minutes later, we crossed Ocean Avenue and made our way back through the throng of shoppers to her stand. She gave the tall young man a kiss on the cheek and sent him on his way.

"You're busy here," I said. "I'd like to pick up Nate if it's all right with you."

She smiled. "Yes, good. He'd like that."

TWENTY-NINE

FBI field headquarters was in the Westwood Federal Building on Wilshire Boulevard just east of the 405 freeway. Built at the height of the Vietnam War, the hulking, nineteen-story tower of steel, glass, and stone stood as a not-so-subtle reminder of the government's authority. I felt nervous just walking toward it through the sprawling parking lot.

I stepped off the elevator on the tenth floor. Pictures of martyred FBI agents dating back to 1925 covered the facing wall. Off to the side in the small reception area, Nate slouched in an oversized black Naugahyde chair. I caught the eye of an agent sitting behind a thick pane of bullet-proof glass and indicated I was there for the old man. He made a shooing motion with the back of his hand. "Take him," he mouthed.

Under the harsh fluorescents, Nate appeared old and frail. The physical contrast between this Nate and the one who roamed free on his mountain was striking, and I wanted to get us out of there before the place sucked all the life out of him.

"I hope you weren't too rough on those guys," I said when we were back in the car.

"Let's go home," he muttered, closing his eyes.

Westbound traffic on Wilshire was heavy, so I decided to take the freeways—a longer route, but under these conditions, faster. I glanced over at Nate now and then. His eyes remained shut; his breath was slow and steady. As the minutes passed, his shoulders dropped and the tension seemed to leave his body. I had the distinct impression that he was recharging himself—not asleep exactly, but in a deeply restful place. He remained in that quiet, cocooned state until we reached the top of Topanga.

"Can you stay for tea?" he asked.

"Sure."

He was already bounding up the hill as I got out of the car. "Good," he shouted, "we've lost time today and there's catching up to do."

I smiled. Nate was himself again.

৵

Back at the house, he went straight for the kitchen and put on a pot of water. I leaned against the doorjamb and watched him go through his well-established ritual—retrieving the mugs and tin container from the cupboard and carefully filling each tea ball with loose tea.

"How much did Heather tell you?" he asked, handing me a steaming mug. "It's licorice root—I think you'll like it."

Given what he'd been through, it didn't seem like a good time to get into too much of that. "She said you sabotaged those helicopters to stop the county from spraying Malathion."

"Uh-huh." He blew into his tea and took a sip. "Well, demonstrations and legal maneuvers weren't getting anywhere. At the time I didn't see any other way."

"I have to say I admire your courage."

"It's only courage when you've got a choice," he replied. He took another sip of tea. "At the time, I saw the Med-fly eradication project as the final proof of our collective, unremitting ignorance. I dismantled those helicopters in a last-ditch effort to prevent us from committing unintentional suicide."

"But you know, they *did* spray and we *are* still here. Maybe you were wrong."

Nate turned toward the kitchen window and stared out at the garden. "I wish I were." It was a long moment before he spoke again. "We've got a few hours of sun yet. Come on, let's stretch our legs."

I took a last gulp of the sweet tea, and Nate grabbed his satchel. He slid a canteen under the tap and handed me the other one to fill. Before I was done, he had shifted into high gear and was out the front door. I slung the canteen's strap over my shoulder and chased after him as he headed toward the trail that led across the field and into the mountains.

"You're not thinking of taking me up that hill again are you?" I yelled.

"Better get used to it," he called back without stopping. "And pick it up. We're losing daylight."

෨෧

Nate paused at the trailhead. "Here's a story that might help you understand why I had to stop those helicopters," he said when I'd caught up with him. "At the end of World War Two, the U.S. government was sitting on stockpiles of surplus nitrates that were no longer needed for bomb manufacture. At the same time, over-farming was draining the Life Force out of this country's topsoil."

He picked up speed as he climbed down into the canyon and, once again started getting a little ahead of me. If I wanted to hear his story, I had to step up my pace, which I'm sure is exactly what he intended.

"They say a little knowledge is a dangerous thing," he continued. "That was certainly true in this case. Ignorant of all the elements that affect Life Force, scientists at the Department of Agriculture in charge of developing a yield-boosting synthetic fertilizer became fixated on one of those elements, nitrogen. Those surplus nitrates were gonna save our crops. As far as the government was concerned, it was a win-win proposition."

Gravel slipped under my feet, but I hurried on, wanting to catch Nate's every word.

"The agriculture bureaucrats pulled large chemical companies into the project, and pretty soon they had something. The fertilizer was distributed to farmers who used it to grow feed for livestock.

"Well, the initial results were spectacular. Feed-crop yields went way up. That meant the price of feed came down, which was good for business. And what was good for business was good for the country. So, more of the synthetic fertilizer was ordered up and put into widespread use."

"So far, it *does* look like a win-win," I said.

"Yes, it did at first," he continued. "But in a few years, ranchers began to report a troubling development: infertility rates were climbing in cattle given the new feed. They wondered if the synthetic fertilizer had anything to do with it and asked the USDA to see if there was a connection. Sure enough, scientists found that something about the fertilizer caused a subtle imbalance in the cattle's hormones—just enough to disrupt fertility."

Nate stopped short. "Now what do you suppose the rational response would be in a situation like that?"

It seemed obvious. "Stop using the fertilizer."

"It's a no-brainer, right? Once it's clear that your actions are causing harm, you stop them."

"Of course."

"Well, the government didn't stop using that fertilizer," he said, shaking his head. "By then, fertilizer manufacturing had become a billion-dollar industry with big lobbyists in Washington. In addition, pulling the fertilizer off the market would have meant a return to lower crop yields and higher food prices. That would be bad for business and bad for the country. No, they needed another solution to the infertility problem."

"More chemicals?"

"Exactly. Large drug companies were called in to help, and pretty soon *they* had something—synthetic hormones. The hormones were added to the cattle's feed to re-establish the animals' hormonal balance. Lo and behold, the livestock began reproducing at an acceptable rate again. Not only was the problem solved, but a lucrative new business was created for the drug companies."

We reached the end of the switchback and turned down the next one. My thighs were burning, and I held my fists down to subtly pound them as I stepped.

"Reminds me of the old saying: two wrongs don't make a right," I said.

Nate spun around. "And what do you think they'd say about three wrongs?"

"What's the third?" I asked, skidding to a stop.

"Do you remember the last time we were in this canyon we spoke about the depletion of Life Force in the soil?"

"Oh, I meant to tell you. I saw it. I saw Life Force in your produce at the farmer's market. It was amazing!"

Nate gave me a faint smile. "That's good...very good," he said, and appeared to allow himself a moment's satisfaction. But he didn't lose his focus. "Now, to that third wrong. Synthetic fertilizer, by definition, is not natural. Synthetic fertilizer doesn't replenish the soil's Life Force—it destroys it."

He put his hand on my arm. "The Life Force you saw in my produce—where did it come from?"

"The soil."

"Correct. The Life Force of crops is only as strong as the Life Force of the soil in which they grow. What did I say weakened crops had to be doused with to survive to harvest?"

"Chemical pesticides."

"Right again. Another billion-dollar industry made necessary by us. Are you starting to see a pattern here?"

"We don't seem to mind messing things up as long as we can make a profit?"

"Yes. We meddle with nature and disrupt the finely calibrated balance that sustains life. But we don't learn from our mistakes and stop meddling. Instead, we attempt to rectify the problems we create with a technological fix. But the fix invariably creates a new problem, requiring another technological solution, which just creates another..."

He started down the trail again.

"It's sheer insanity," he continued, his voice sounding angry now, "but it seems perfectly rational to us. We refuse to recognize that there's a limit to the amount of jerry-rigging the Earth will tolerate before its precarious life-sustaining balance is lost for good."

We crunched along without talking for the next few minutes. I wasn't sweating hard, but I took it as a bad sign that I was sweating at all on the downhill leg of the trek. My body didn't seem to know basic protocol for a hike, like "downhill is the *easy* part."

When we arrived at the bottom, Nate sat on a creek-side boulder and pulled his satchel onto his lap. I found a flat rock and tried to make myself comfortable. "I brought us some fuel for our little hike," he said, pulling out four strips of jerky and offering a couple to me.

As I reached for them, our shared dream came back to mind. Compared to what we'd done then, the impending climb seemed like what it was—recreation, not torture. Maybe someday it would feel like that too. The two of us ate in silence for awhile. I stared into the clear water churning past the rocks at my feet.

"Nate, what you said about the pesticides. It reminded me of something I read—that there are thousands of them used in this country."

"Close to nine thousand, I believe. Some are more harmful than others, but nearly all of them have a negative impact beyond their target species."

"You must have felt pretty strongly about Malathion to go after those helicopters."

He took a bite of jerky, chewed for awhile, and chased it with a drink from his canteen. I sailed a twig into the stream and we both watched until it disappeared.

"We eat by the grace of nature," he finally said, letting the sound of the rushing creek underline his point. "Long and short of it is this: if we don't stop spraying Malathion, we're all going to starve to death."

Hearing Nate say those words with that "voice of God" made the hairs on the back of my neck bristle.

"You're familiar with pollination, aren't you?" he asked.

"Sure," I replied.

"Think about it," he said. "Every fruit and vegetable and a fair amount of the feed crops we grow for our livestock require a pollinator to carry the male pollen grain from one plant's stamen to the female pistil of another, where fertilization occurs."

"Right, plant sex."

"And what creature makes all that plant sex possible?"

"The guys with the stingers," I said. "Bees."

Nate finished his last bit of jerky and stood up. Break over.

"Malathion kills bees. It's especially good at it. Bees aren't its target species, of course, but the result is the same." He started across the creek, quick-stepping from rock to rock. "No bees, no pollination. No pollination, no food. No food, no us." He sounded oddly calm, as though he were narrating the end of some *other* planet.

"Jesus, we're not that close, are we?"

"Since Malathion was introduced in 1950, bee populations have declined by 90 percent. At the rate we're going, it won't be long."

"That's completely fucked, pardon my French. Who let this happen? Isn't anyone at the EPA paying attention?"

"Son, this problem wasn't caused by inattention at some governmental agency."

He reached the other side and turned. His voice punched right through the hiss of the stream.

"When I sabotaged those helicopters, I was naïve enough to think that the problem began and ended with the collapse of the bee population. But it runs much deeper, and even a thousand acts of civil disobedience aren't going to change things. From the moment we disconnected from the biofield and put ourselves in charge of this planet, we have waged war on the natural world and plundered her resources to satisfy our appetite for food and fuel."

I gingerly stepped to the streambed, hoping to avoid the inevitable, but one slip and I was in up to the ankle. I splashed the rest of the way across, and Nate watched with a smile. "You'll be all right. It's just water."

Almost as if to distract me, he resumed his lesson. "Look what we've managed to do running things on our own without that link to the biofield. We've altered the Earth's atmosphere, and her temperature is rising like a fever. The heat is melting her ice caps and glaciers and sucking the water out of her soil. Pretty soon, floods and droughts will make entire regions uninhabitable. When that happens, man won't be the only species scrambling to survive, and the illusion of control will vanish. Order will devolve into chaos, and nature will rise and wage a war of her own. Don't bet on us winning that one."

I was still wringing out the leg of my pants as Nate started up the path on the other side, his voice ringing off the rocks.

"By the way, congratulations on seeing Life Force. You took a big step in the right direction today."

"Thanks. That was really something."

He turned and gave me a proud nod. "Well," he cleared his throat, "Let's keep moving. I'll see you up at Two Gulls."

"Two Gulls?"

"I've renamed the summit in honor of the pair of seagulls that visited us the last time we were there."

He bent to gather a handful of dirt and small stones.

"This earth is not our property, to do with as we please, but must be shared with all living things. Giving places and people animal names is an old tradition that reminds us of that fact and of our oneness with nature."

"Okay," I said, my mind still back with the bees, melted glaciers, and the water squishing out of my soles. "See you at Two Gulls."

THIRTY

The trail to the top wound in and out of the shade of live oaks and sycamores, but even the low rays of the sun were intense. My feet were still damp, but at least they'd cooled me off a little on the climb. Even so, I was out of breath and sweating hard. As I approached the summit, Nate was lying on his back, hands behind his head, communing with the afternoon sky. I willed my aching legs to transport me the short distance between us, then collapsed straight down—a perfect one-point landing on my ass.

"This mountain…just might be…the death of me," I managed to say between gasps for air.

"Or the cure," Nate replied, keeping his eyes on a circling hawk. "Take a moment to catch your breath, and then tell me what you've learned so far about leading an authentic life."

I rolled onto my side, rested my cheek on my open palm and inhaled deeply. There was sage in the air, a dry spiciness that I'd begun to notice on the way up.

"Let's see…I've learned that I have to stop eating unconsciously, get rid of junk food in my diet, and feed my body food that's high in Life Force."

"What else have you learned?"

"What else…I've learned that I need to eat with an intention to receive the nutrients food has to offer me. And you said that having unlimited access to food can cause garbage to accumulate in me—so it's a good idea to take a few days off every once in awhile. If I drink fresh juice and give my digestive system a break, my body gets a chance to clean house—not that 'cleaning house' is the most fun project in the world. But I guess it gets easier if you don't have as much gunk to get rid of."

Nate turned toward me and propped himself up on his elbow. "What else have you learned?"

My thighs throbbed, so I sat up and rubbed them. Taking Nate's quiz was at least making it clear that I *had* been learning things I wouldn't soon forget. "Okay, I've learned that I'm totally out of shape, but my body craves activity and physical challenge. That was a new one on me. And, I've got to tell you, right now that 'challenge' hurts like hell."

"Inertia's a bitch," he said. "You'll get over it." He pushed himself up and sat cross-legged, laying his hands on his thighs, palms up. "Lucky for you the next lesson requires no physical exertion. Here, face me and sit like this."

I forced myself up.

"Now close your eyes and be still."

I shut them.

"What do you notice?"

I raised one eyelid. "Is this another test? There's not a *fourth* level of awareness, is there?"

214

"No, this is not a test. Now, shut that eye and tell me what comes to your attention."

With my eyes closed, I immediately noticed the sound of dry leaves blowing past, the smell of sage and sea air, and the ocean breeze on my skin. I reported these things to Nate.

"Good," he said. "Sensory information—that's the first level. What does your body have to say for itself?"

"My legs feel stiff, my sit-bones hurt," I said. "That ache under my right shoulder is back, and it's moving into my neck."

"Physical symptoms. That's the second level. Stay with it."

I adjusted my position to get more comfortable, and my attention was instantly drawn to a swarm of thoughts buzzing in my head. I took a deep breath to clear them away, but they refused to stop.

"Pretty busy up there, isn't it?" Nate said, as if he knew just what was going on.

"Like Grand Central Station. No, busier."

"That chatter in your head is a reflection of the stress your body is carrying, forty-one years' worth. You might not notice it during the day when your senses are distracting you. But it's always there. In our first meeting, you told me that your thoughts make it difficult for you to fall asleep. Remember?"

"Yeah, unless I'm totally exhausted that chatter can keep me up for quite awhile."

"That's your stress talking. When you go to bed and close down sensory input, the mind begins to quiet to allow you to fall asleep; this signals the body to quiet too. As it relaxes, the body's first instinct is to throw off stress, which it considers toxic. But here's the rub: a thought is the corresponding response in the quieted mind to the release of stress by the body. That buzzing in your head is a pretty good barometer of the amount of stress you're carrying."

"I don't feel *that* stressed."

Nate chucked. "And a fish doesn't know it's wet. Modern life is saturated with stress. It's unavoidable. Traffic jams, parking tickets, money worries, pressure to get ahead, troubles at work, time constraints, competition, marriage, divorce, and underneath it all, the constant drone of unsettling news from around the world. Hell, I live by myself on top of a mountain, and you saw what happened to me today."

He put both his hands on my shoulders. "You're a new father, and for all practical purposes, you're out of work. If stress *were* water, you'd be up to your eyeballs in it."

I could feel my neck and shoulders tensing up at the words "out of work." The rest of me tightened too. Nate must've noticed. He handed me my canteen. "Speaking of water, we should have some," he said.

We each took a few swallows.

"Back when you and I were chasing mastodons, stressful events didn't last long. Run-ins with wild animals or enemies would activate the fight-or-flight response, causing a temporary surge of cortisol and epinephrine, stress hormones the body produces that improve its ability to fight or run like hell. Regardless of the outcome, the event was over fast, and cortisol and epinephrine levels would soon return to normal. There's no doubt, this response served mankind well for hundreds of thousands of years.

"But the moment we turned our back on the biofield, the nature of our stress changed dramatically. It no longer came in short bursts, but got woven into the fabric of our daily lives. And the hormones it generated began to flow nonstop.

The results on the human body have not been pretty: fatigue, chronic aches and pains, anxiety, depression, weakened immunity, accelerated aging, heart disease, even cancer."

He screwed the cap back on his canteen. "Stress can definitely kill you. The diseases it doesn't cause, it contributes to. Don't underestimate it. Get everything else right, but ignore your stress and it will find a way to take you down single-handedly."

I picked up a pebble and aimed at a tree, missing wildly.

"Then I'm probably screwed," I said, forcing a laugh.

He looked at me almost sympathetically. "Or you could learn to deal with it. One thing I can tell you is that the body can only release stress when sensory input is minimized and the mind is quiet."

"Okay."

"So, what are you going to do, knowing that?"

"Sleep more?"

"Not a bad guess. Sleep is designed for rejuvenation and regeneration—critical processes that keep us young—but it was never meant to process the exorbitant amount of stress bombarding us in the modern world. Charge it with that task, and you sabotage the works. Aging accelerates, stress accumulates—not exactly the recipe for a long and healthy life."

"Like I said—I'm screwed. All I know how to do is write songs, and I quit *that* to hike around with you. I'm okay as long as I don't think about it, but it's hard not to, you know?" My little volley of pebbles made soft clicks as they hit the ground.

"Listen, son. I'm going to assume you're looking for a solution and that you're not interested in giving up."

I nodded.

"It's simple, then. Instead of expecting sleep to deal with your stress, you must find another time of day to quiet your mind."

"That's what you were doing in the car, isn't it?"

"Those boys at the FBI were pretty hard on me, and you saw the shape I was in when you picked me up. I'll show you what I did to unload all that stress."

He sat straight up. "Before we try it, there's something else I want to tell you. This technique delivers a second-ary benefit that's just as important as the primary one. It's clear you're ready to re-establish your connection to the Self. You proved that when you saw Life Force today. But remember, the Self speaks in a very soft voice. It can't compete with the clatter of thoughts your stress is generat-ing. You'll only hear it in the quiet spaces between those thoughts."

I shut my eyes for a moment and then opened them again. "Easy for you to say. There *is* no quiet space between my thoughts."

Nate smiled. "Not yet. First you have to excavate the stress that generates them."

Nate scanned the afternoon sky and then his eyes fell back on me. "Now, do you want to talk the subject to death or are you ready to learn something?"

"Let's do it."

༄

"Are you comfortable?" he asked.

I shifted my position slightly. "Yes, fine."

"Close your eyes." He paused for several seconds. "Allow those thoughts to play in your mind. Make no attempt to control them. Let them come…and go."

Letting go was not so easy. I was used to taking charge of my thoughts and steering them one way or another.

"Let them come, and let them go," he repeated. "Just watch what's going on in there as if you were an outsider, looking in. As you do, allow your breath to occur naturally. Don't try to control it in any conscious way."

With that suggestion, my mind locked on my breath. *Breathe. Breathe. Breathe!* My eyes snapped open. "You might as well say, 'Don't think of an elephant,' or 'Don't think of the color red.' If you tell me not to, of course I'm going to think about it."

"There's a difference between awareness and control. Until I mentioned it, had you thought about breathing today?"

"No."

"And yet, you did breathe."

"Of course."

"The fact that breath happens without conscious control is what makes it an effective mantra. Attempting to control it makes that impossible."

"Wait. I thought a mantra was a sound, like *Om* or something."

"Actually," he said, "you can think of it as the key to quieting your mind. As amazing as the mind is, it can only focus on one thing at a time. In the meditation I'm going to teach you, the mantra works by giving the mind something other than surface thought to focus on. This allows the mind to turn inward to deeper and quieter levels of consciousness, which is its instinctive desire."

"Meditation? Jesus, Nate, I'm not ready for some religious thing."

"It's not religion, son. Now close your eyes."

Resistance was futile. I closed them.

"Allow thoughts to come and go," he said softly, "and let your breath occur, naturally."

It took awhile, but I was finally able to mentally "step back" and let my thoughts and breathing happen on their own.

"Now," he continued, "begin to favor the breath as a focal point. Focus on whatever aspect of your breathing draws your attention—the rise and fall of your chest or belly—the flow of air through your nostrils."

I focused on the air moving into my nose, but was quickly distracted by a flurry of random thoughts. *I wonder what Merry's making for dinner...got to find a body shop to repair the Volvo...I wish I had a pillow to sit on...did I lock the car?* If you'd asked me what I was doing, I would've said, "Just thinking."

"Invariably," Nate continued, his voice even softer now, "your attention will be drawn away from the breath and begin to follow a thought or a feeling. This sort of distraction is normal. It's actually an indication that the process is working. Remember, each time the body releases stress, the mind responds with a thought. So whenever you notice that you are no longer observing your breathing, it's important that you gently and without judgment bring your mind's attention back to the breath. This will allow your mind to quiet again, if only for a moment, and let your body throw off more stress."

Then he stopped talking.

I watched the air moving through my nose, cool on inhalation, warm on exhalation. When I noticed I was thinking,

I turned my focus back to my breath. I repeated that process over and over, and eventually I became so relaxed I was unaware of my physical body. I lost track of time. At one point, I must have fallen asleep, because the next thing I knew, my head had dropped halfway to my knees. I pulled myself upright and watched my breath for another minute or so before Nate spoke again.

"Now, allow thoughts to come and go again without putting any special emphasis on tracking the breath. Wait about a minute and then slowly open your eyes."

As I observed the contents of my mind, I noticed a slight pressure building, which felt like the seed of a headache. But the moment I put my attention on it the sensation vanished. I took a deep breath and opened my eyes.

"How was that?" he asked.

"I feel like I've just had a mini-vacation."

The energy between us was very peaceful, very calm. The profound shift I saw in him after he zoned out on the way home from the FBI made sense now.

"Good, then you won't mind going on that vacation on a regular basis."

"Not at all."

"This method gives the body a chance to rest at a very deep level—for me, one session can be the equivalent of several hours' sleep. You'll be eliminating stress, and taking regular trips to where the Self resides."

"That space between thoughts."

"The third level of awareness. With a little practice, you should have no trouble receiving and transmitting the biofield's positive energy."

"Transmitting?"

"Once you are in touch with the Self and the limitless knowledge it has access to, your thinking is going to change. You will live more instinctually, and you'll be more mindful, more appreciative of all of nature's gifts. You will also be able to direct positive energy anywhere within the biofield."

"How do I do that?"

"Think good thoughts about something, admire it, sing it a song. Whatever is on the receiving end will benefit."

"That's kind of woo-woo stuff," I said.

"That's quantum physics. The details are beyond the scope of these lessons. Suffice it to say that the energy you put out has a direct impact on the world around you. Sing to a plant, and it will grow healthier. Admire a flower, and its colors will become more brilliant. Appreciate the graceful flight of two seagulls, and they will soar higher."

"Love the world, and the world will love you back, huh?"

"Is that so hard to fathom?" he asked with a kind smile. "When we feel love for something we are, in effect, sending it a gift of positive energy. If that love is well placed, it is always returned in some way." He stood up and brushed the dirt off the seat of his jeans. "Do you have any idea what love is?"

"I know when I'm feeling it."

"Feelings, yes, but what causes those feelings? What's behind them? What is love in its purest form?"

"I couldn't tell you," I said, getting to my feet.

"The harmonious flow of energy that sustains everything," he said. "*That* is love." He ran his thumb down his jawline and thought for a moment. "We protect what we love, don't we?"

"Yes."

"Why?"

"So it'll survive."

"Because?"

"Because when we love something, we don't want to live without it."

He turned to face me. "There are some things you wouldn't want to live without and others you couldn't live without. Which would you protect more fiercely?"

"Things I *couldn't* live without," I said.

Nate picked up a stick, drew a circle in the dirt, then a much smaller one a few feet from the first. He poked his stick at the smaller circle. "You live on this tiny blue dot, orbiting in cold and empty space, ninety-three million miles from the sun. The balance of elements that permits life on this little dot is exceedingly fragile. Altered even slightly, by God's hand or ours, it could quickly become uninhabitable." He let the stick drop. "How much do you love your home, and what are you willing to do to protect the life you have here?"

"Until I met you I can honestly say I never thought much about that."

Nate smiled. "Love and life are inseparable. Love created your daughter. The demonstration of that love keeps her alive. Love produced the life in my garden and orchard. If I ever stopped expressing my love for those plants, stopped tending them, they would wither and die."

He scooped up his satchel and swung it over his shoulder. "When something depends on you for its survival, it's not enough to merely feel love for it. Your actions must reflect that love."

"I can see that."

"Well, for better or worse, the Earth's creatures are our children, her forests and fields are our garden." He turned and took a few steps down the trail.

"Wait a second," I said. "Did you just say that love is the harmonious flow of energy that sustains everything?"

He stopped but didn't look back. "Uh-huh."

"But the biofield sustains everything."

"That's right."

"So are you saying that the energy flowing through the biofield is...love?"

"I can't think of a better name for it." He turned, held my gaze for a moment, and then started down the mountain. "Let's go. It's almost dark." As I followed, he called back to me. "This evening, ask your wife if she minds your spending a couple of days at my place. Do you own a sleeping bag?"

"I think so."

"Good, if she gives you the okay, bring it with you tomorrow morning with a toothbrush and a change of clothes."

THIRTY-ONE

"This Nate must be really good," Merry remarked later that night, as she pulled her old sleeping bag out of a box in our garage. "You, camping out. Whoa! That's a big step for a guy who thinks roughing it is staying in a hotel without room service."

"He didn't say anything about camping out. There's one bed, and I think he's going to put me on the floor."

"Well, if he has something more exotic in mind..." she smiled broadly. "Get him to take a photo of you if you wind up sleeping outside. That would be priceless. Anyhow, you'll be fine. I'll pack you some extra clothes, just in case."

"Okay, I'm a wimp. What can I say?"

She dropped the sleeping bag and threw her arms around my waist. "Maybe the 'old' Sam was."

I gave her a long kiss. "And the 'new' Sam?"

"Hmmm," she cooed. "I like this one."

"Glad you approve." I kissed her again. "I better take a shower and get to bed. I want to be at Nate's early tomorrow."

Merry checked her watch. "Ten o'clock? You *are* a changed man."

"Yeah, well, it looks like it's going to be a tough day." I pulled her closer. "Say, lady, care to join me?"

Merry didn't wait until I was out of the shower. She stepped in behind me as I was washing my hair. We soaped each other up and made love right there. Afterward, we lay in bed talking until I couldn't keep my eyes open anymore.

∾

A solitary star pushed a pinprick of light into a vast, black space. That light intensified, and I felt myself racing toward it at tremendous speed. I shot past an enormous, cold planet into more engulfing emptiness. The star grew brighter as I gazed through a gigantic field of asteroids. I had just re-entered our solar system from somewhere deep in the cosmos.

Continuing on, I sailed the solar wind as comets, their dust tails glowing behind them, streaked away from the sun. On the other side of Mars, a tiny blue dot appeared. Aided by some internal guidance system, I slowed and banked toward it. The dot grew into a sphere, and soon I was hovering half-way between the moon and our brilliant blue-and-white marbled planet.

I stayed suspended there, in the Earth's gentle pull, and marveled at the graceful movement of its continents and oceans as they revolved into sunlight and back into shadow. I could feel the miracle of it, this living, breathing world floating in infinite, lifeless space.

Then, with a single thought, I swooped down, counterclockwise, around the nightside of the planet. I passed over the dark Pacific to the western edge of North America, then down the coast and across Santa Monica Bay as the hint of daybreak, in orange and blue pastels, glowed on the eastern horizon.

∽

I felt someone shaking my arm. "Rise and shine," Merry said brightly.

I cracked one eyelid and checked the time—6:05. "You're awfully perky this morning," I answered.

"Yeah, I feel good. We should get to bed early more often."

I sat up and blinked open both eyes. Merry was pulling clothes out of the dresser and putting them in my canvas overnight bag. "I packed your thermal underwear and a sweater in case you end up sleeping under the stars." She suppressed a giggle.

"Bite your tongue." *Stars...I'll have to tell Nate about the dream.*

I shaved and dressed while Merry made us breakfast—scrambled eggs and tomato slices. "No toast?" she asked.

"You know, since that juice thing I did, I just haven't been hungry for starchy carbs. I'm gonna see how I feel if I go light on them." The truth was, when Maggie called me a carbohydrate addict, it touched a nerve. I didn't like the idea of being addicted to anything.

"It's inspiring, these changes you're making," Merry said. "Maybe I'll pull down my veggie cookbooks."

The sound of Zoë stirring in her crib cut short our conversation.

"I've got the dishes," I said, rising from the table.

Merry stood and gave me a kiss. "Say, Dad, this will be the first night you're spending away from your daughter."

"Yeah."

"Well, call if you get homesick. But I think it'll be fun. Who knows, maybe you'll get in touch with your inner Euell Gibbons."

"Make fun if you want," I said. "But anything's possible." I found myself humming as I did the dishes, and when they were done, I collected my gear, kissed my girls, and headed for Topanga.

∽

"I'm in the garden," Nate hollered as I approached the house. I dropped my bags in the living room and walked out to the landing at the top of the back stairs. Nate stood at the plot of ground where we had recently spread the compost. He held a tray of something green. "Grab that last flat of seedlings, would you?"

I picked it up from the table at the entrance to the orchard, and as I carried it across the garden, counted eighteen baby plants in three rows. I set the flat of seedlings down next to several others.

"Did you eat?" he asked.

"Yes, sir."

"Did you meditate?"

228

"Meditate? Well…"

"It's best to do that first thing in the morning, before anything else. Otherwise, you'll have to try to squeeze it into your schedule, which usually doesn't work."

"Okay, sorry."

"Don't be. Here." He handed me a wooden stake with a string attached to it. "Shove that into the ground right there in the corner of the garden."

I tried it with the heel of my hand but it wouldn't budge. I used my body weight to push it in with my foot.

He walked the string across the width of the garden and secured it in the opposite corner with another stake. I noticed that the string was marked evenly, about every two feet, with black ink.

"Those marks show the distance between rows," he said, picking up another pair of stakes attached to a much longer string. "Take this to the far end, and we'll line up the first row."

Nate planted his stake. "Okay, make sure she's parallel to the edge, and set her tight."

The plot of ground was probably thirty feet from end to end. I eyeballed the line as best I could, pulled the string taut and pushed the wooden stake into the soil. "That's good. Come get the next one."

We repeated the process five times. Nate secured his end first, then I set the string parallel to the last one and used my heel to secure a stake at the opposite end of the garden. The entire procedure took less than fifteen minutes.

"That was fun," I said, brushing a little dirt off my hands.

Nate handed me a trowel. "Glad you enjoyed yourself. Those six strings we set lengthwise are marked every eighteen inches. We're going to plant a seedling at each one of those marks, two rows of broccoli, two of cauliflower and two of cabbage.

I started doing the math. *Thirty-six seedlings of each, times three...*

"There are a hundred and eight. Fretting about it won't get them in the ground any quicker." He knelt next to one of the flats. "Have a seat."

I found a patch of grass and sat down on it.

"You want to tell me anything?"

"Tell you?"

"Anything of interest happen last night?"

"You mean my dream?"

"Oh, you had a dream," he said, with exaggerated surprise, making it clear he already knew. "Tell me about it."

I described the whole thing in as much detail as I could remember.

"What do you make of it?" he asked.

"It struck me how infinitely cold and empty space is and how lucky I am to be alive at all."

"Anything else?"

"The Earth was gorgeous, no question about it."

"And?"

I thought for a moment and shrugged.

"You said you hovered in space for quite awhile, watching the continents and oceans revolve from light into dark, from day into night."

"Yes, that's right."

"Light and dark, day and night—therein lies the message. And, as it happens, that is the subject of your final lesson."

He pulled a flat toward him with the letters 'BRO' written on its side. "But first, we've got work to do." He scooped a seedling out with his trowel and placed it in his hand. "Snip off the bottom pair of leaves like this." He pinched each leaf between his thumb and forefinger and gently removed it. "See this crook here in the stem? They'll all have it. Plant the seedlings deep enough to cover that crook. When you've got it in the ground, make sure to press the soil firmly around its base. Any questions?"

I shook my head.

"Good." He handed me the little seedling. "You take the broccoli."

My experience with planting vegetables was limited to taking overripe potatoes that had sprouted eyes and burying them in the backyard as a kid. I felt clumsy getting the seedlings out of the flat unscathed, and I was all thumbs trying to remove their tiny leaves, then plant them at just the right depth. My progress was painfully slow. By the time I transplanted the first row of seedlings and was pulling the second flat into position, Nate had all the cauliflower in the ground and was moving on to the cabbage.

"Ever heard of Carolus Linnaeus?" he asked, retrieving the new flat.

"I vaguely remember the name from grade school science," I said, "but I couldn't tell you much about him."

"Let me refresh your memory. He lived over two hundred years ago. He was a Swedish biologist, one of the first men to study the order of nature." Nate set the flat down and scooped out a cabbage seedling. "This fellow Linnaeus observed that the blossoms of various flowers open at specific times of the day. For instance, morning glories open at six in the morning, dandelions at seven. The California poppy opens at ten, passion flower at noon and evening primrose at six in the evening."

He pinched the bottom pair of leaves off a seedling. "I'll give you one guess what time the four o'clock plant opens its petals."

I stood, careful not to tweak my lower back. "Can you give me a hint?"

He gave me an exasperated look.

"You're serious?" I said. "Flowers can actually tell you what time it is?"

"For two hundred years, people have been turning circular gardens into living clocks that do just that."

He wiped his forehead with the sleeve of his denim shirt. "So, young man, why do you imagine I bother telling you this?"

I shrugged.

"I'll give you a hint. Your dream and flower clocks have something in common—a powerful, fundamental principle of natural law we humans once obeyed without question, but now ignore at our peril." Nate set the cabbage seedling in the ground and carefully gathered the soil around its base. "Think about it while you finish planting that row and you can tell me what you've come up with while we make lunch."

THIRTY-TWO

I transplanted the second row of broccoli and got up to trail Nate around the garden as he collected vegetables for lunch.

"I think I have something," I said. "The flowers in the clock open at different times of the day in response to the changing light. That's the connection to my dream, isn't it?"

Nate dropped a couple of carrots into a basket and handed it to me. "And what principle of natural law do you suppose that phenomenon represents?"

"Something about the sun."

"The sun and what?"

"And its effect on life."

We moved over to a patch of lettuce. "Rhythm," he said, using his pocketknife to harvest a half dozen mature leaves. "Everything from atoms to planetary systems has a rhythm to it." He laid the leaves in the basket. "Grab a cucumber from that trellis, would you?" He handed me the knife and pointed across the garden. "The rhythm of life on Earth is set by the planet's rotation, the varying times of sunrise and sunset and consequent cycles of light and dark. Understanding the importance of this rhythm and synchronizing your life to it is your final lesson."

I found a nice-looking cucumber and pulled it from under the scratchy leaves of the vine. "Rhythm, huh?" In my mind, I launched into "I've Got Rhythm," using the cuke as a microphone, and threw in some Fred Astaire-ish moves.

Not privy to my inner performance, Nate continued. "Specifically, we're talking about circadian rhythm, from the Latin, *circa dies*, which means 'around a day.'" He turned toward the house. "You make the salad, son. I'll broil us up a couple of chicken breasts. A friend of mine raises some very tasty grain-fed, free-range birds."

Back in the kitchen, I washed and chopped the vegetables. Nate put the chicken under the broiler, and the lesson continued.

"According to Charles Darwin, the phenomenon of flowers opening at different times of the day reflects each plant's specific needs for survival—getting just the right amount and intensity of sun and being open for business when a pollinator is most likely to visit." Nate reached into the cupboard, rummaging through the small jars and cans inside and extracting a tin of paprika. "Do you think this is something a plant does consciously?"

"Plants don't have brains, so it's gotta be automatic."

"Right, the plant's biorhythm, which determines the opening and closing of its flowers, is calibrated by the Earth's rotation."

Nate pulled out the chicken and gave it a quick sprinkle. "Let's say we were able to grant the power of free will to the morning glory. Now, instead of automatically opening its petals at six a.m. to attract insects that help it reproduce, and closing them again at noon to avoid overexposure to the sun's radiation, each morning glory is free to decide for itself how it *wants* to behave.

"With this newfound ability, some of the glories might choose to open when it's dark to see what they've been missing all night. Others may decide they'd rather be 'afternoon glories' and refuse to open their funnel-shaped blossoms until the sun is at its strongest. A few might be content to continue their long-standing tradition of opening at six and closing at noon, because they trust that nature had a good reason to cause them to behave that way in the first place."

I swept some chopped carrots into a wooden salad bowl. "I'm going to take a wild guess and say the ones that altered their behavior didn't do so well."

"Good guess. The glories that opened at night ended up shut during the day when insects that could pollinate them were making their rounds. The glories that insisted on opening their petals in the heat of the midday sun suffered irreparable radiation damage."

"So, you're saying that the only morning glories that would thrive are the ones that use their free will to behave as if they had none at all." I was getting hungry and started using the "one for me, one for the salad" technique with the cucumber, picking slices off the cutting board and beginning to munch. "I always thought free will was such a big deal, something that separates humans from all other creatures. Judging from this little fairy tale of yours, you're not a big fan."

"On the contrary, free will is a real gift. But it must be used judiciously. You *could* eat nothing but donuts for breakfast, lunch, and dinner and sit around on your ass all day playing the guitar. As a human, you have those options. But I think you've learned that your choices and decisions must be tempered with a healthy respect for nature's original plan for you and a willingness to remain mindful of your body's physical needs and limitations." He glanced into the half-empty wooden bowl. "You plan to finish up that salad sometime today?"

"Oh, right," I said, turning back to the untouched lettuce. "I'll admit I was clueless about what I need when we started, but I've got a pretty good handle on all that now."

"You think so?"

"Yes."

"What time did you get to bed last night?"

"About ten o'clock. I wanted to be here early."

"So, your normal bedtime is…"

"Somewhere between eleven-thirty and one, but it can be later if I'm in the studio and on a roll."

"And you consider getting to bed in the middle of the night a wise use of the free will nature bestowed on you?"

"I'm no plant, Nate. Yeah, I think when I'm working, it's a great use of free will."

Nate looked up from the meat he was flipping on the broiler pan. "And that's where you're wrong. Your sad physical condition and lost creativity can be attributed to any one of your poor habits, not least of which is your insistence on staying up to all hours. As things stand, you don't have the sense God gave a morning glory.

"Think about it. When you and I were going after mastodons, wasn't the hunt tough enough in the light of day? If our tribe had insisted on hunting at night, do you think we would have survived to pass on our DNA?"

"No, but I don't see any mastodons headed this way, do you?"

"This may come as a shock," Nate continued unfazed, "but man did not evolve as a nocturnal creature. Nature gave us none of the specialized senses required for functioning well in the dark. As a result, we evolved to be active during the day and inactive at night."

"But we had the brains to invent light bulbs."

"Bulbs or no bulbs, the energy in here"—Nate tapped my chest—"ebbs and flows with the same clocklike precision as that of a flower, and for the same reason: to ensure your survival.

"During the day, that energy is meant to be directed out into the world. But at night, the seventy-five trillion cells in this body, responding to biorhythms eons old, compel you to rest and channel your energy inward to accomplish the vitally important tasks associated with repair and maintenance.

"These cycles are nonnegotiable. They *cannot* and *will not* be altered to accommodate your personal agenda. When you use the free will nature gave you to stay awake half the night, she makes no adjustments to compensate for your error, and you wind up denying your body the opportunity to keep itself in good working order. Instead of waking up refreshed and in good repair, you struggle out of bed exhausted and a little older than necessary.

"Don't confuse free will with a free ride. Just because you *can* do something, doesn't mean you *should*. And if doing that something puts you outside the boundaries nature intended for you, you will surely pay the price."

The price. He meant the way I used to crawl into the day after a typical late night. The headaches and backaches. The ubiquitous Pepto Bismol bottle standing sentinel at my bedside. That surely sucked. But my mind was still arguing.

"The thing is, I don't want to pay the *other* price," I told him. "I do my best work at night—well, did anyway. I don't know if I'm willing to lose that."

"Sam," Nate said, looking me in the eye, "I haven't met a person yet that didn't have a good excuse for staying up too late. But nature doesn't care whether you feel justified depriving your body the proper rest. Use your free will to do whatever you want, just be aware that there are consequences to applying it unwisely. You have to decide how long you want to live and how healthy you want to be. It's your choice."

He arranged our chicken on a pair of plates and carried them over to the table. "I'm ready if you are. Let's eat."

The food was delicious, probably made more so by the morning's hard work and the slow, silent pace of the meal. Food really does taste better when you chew it, I thought. That was still a surprise. So was the chicken, which was oddly more flavorful than what I was used to, even without KFC's extra spicy coating.

When we finished, I stood to clear our plates from the table.

"So, okay, if I'm gonna be a good little flower, what time should I go to bed?"

"That all depends on the kind of flower you are." He followed me into the kitchen. "I'll wash, you dry."

"Okay, I'll bite," I said. "What kind of flower am I?"

238

"Don't know. Humans require anywhere from eight to ten hours of rest a night, depending on how hard they work, their genetics, and the season, of course."

"Depending on the season?"

"Unlike morning glories that open and close at the same time year-round, our body clocks are reset every morning by the rising and setting sun to keep us in sync with the planet's available light. At this latitude, daylight lasts four and a half hours longer in June than in December. As diurnal creatures, we naturally need more sleep in the winter, when the nights are long, than we do in the summer, when they're short." He handed me a clean, wet plate, and I pulled a towel off a hook on the sideboard to dry it. "Think about this: Every diurnal animal on Earth, save man, limits its activity to the hours of available light."

"Wait. Diurnal—what is that, anyway?"

"As opposed to nocturnal—I'm sure you've noticed how much harder it is to get out of bed on a dark winter morning than on a summer morning when the bedroom is flooded with sunlight."

"I'm almost never up that early, but I'll take your word."

Nate let out a sigh. "You're never up that early because you stay awake too late. Your body instinctively knows how to keep you synchronized with the circadian rhythm of this planet. If you want to make the most of this life, you'll pay attention and rest when it tells you to."

I polished up the last glass, and Nate and I went back to the garden. We'd be pruning the fruit trees for the rest of the day, he said. Well, he'd be pruning. I was consigned to gathering the clippings and hauling them down to the compost bins. It was a long, mindless task, and I was more than ready to stop when, at about four o'clock, Nate threw his garden gloves into the wheelbarrow.

"We've got just enough time to get washed and up to Two Gulls," he said. "And unless you're planning on carrying your gear all the way, I'll need to rig a backpack for you."

I could see myself teetering down the steep ravine and up to Two Gulls. That trip was hard enough with *no* gear. I stood next to the compost, thinking about how I was going to break it to him that I wasn't going. Nate spoke before I could.

"Humans have been sleeping outdoors for hundreds of thousands of years. I think you'll survive one night. Besides, if you want to know what kind of flower you are, the answer waits on top of that mountain."

I stood like a helpless little kid as he arranged my stuff on a pack frame and helped me heave it to my shoulders. Then we crossed the adjacent field of dry brush, painted gold by the low rays of the sun, and headed down into the shadowed ravine. Fully loaded, the backpack was just heavy enough to throw off my center of gravity. As I'd feared, I came close to toppling over while negotiating a couple of the switchbacks.

When we reached the creek at the bottom, Nate set down his pack and pulled a cloth sack from a side compartment. He untied its cord and reached in.

"Suppertime," he said, "hold out your hands."

He deposited about a dozen almonds in my cupped palms. "There are vegetable sticks too if you're interested."

"Yes, I'm interested. I'm starving. Is this it?"

"You've already learned *what* to eat and *how* to eat. Now you must learn how *much* to eat and *when*." He stepped closer and rested his hand on my back. "This body of yours is a twenty-four-hour-a-day operation, charged with accomplishing innumerable, complex tasks to stay youthful and disease-free. In its wisdom, it directs its energy into different systems at different times of the day to ensure there's enough to go around."

He patted my head. "Are you getting this?"

I started in on my almond "dinner" and gave him a thumbs-up. *Bon appetite!*

"Converting food into fuel and the raw material your body needs for repair takes ten times more energy than any other internal process. If you're smart you'll challenge your digestive system with that task when it has the wherewithal to get the job done."

"When is that?"

Nate opened his canteen and took a quick drink. "Digestive energy peaks around lunchtime and ebbs as the sun goes down, which coincidentally, is when the body is getting ready to use the nutrients that were digested and absorbed earlier for repairs. If the body is forced to process a big dinner, there simply isn't enough energy left for maintenance." He slipped his backpack on and stepped across the creek. "So if you're interested in getting old fast, eat too much too late."

On the climb up, I got the distinct impression that Nate was purposefully slowing his pace to keep an eye on me in case I fell over. But the scenery kept me distracted from my physical discomfort, and I managed to stay on my feet for the entire ascent. My legs were heavy, but they kept moving.

When we reached Two Gulls, we dropped our packs beside the drawing of the Sun and Earth Nate had made in the dirt the day before, and I followed him up a bit farther to a rock outcropping on the west-facing side of the mountain. The burnt-orange sun sat on the horizon, and the shadows grew long in Topanga Canyon. I lowered my eyes. On the crest of a hill a few hundred feet below us, Nate's house and garden stood, deep green and luminous.

"Let's go," he said, "I want to finish this lesson before dark."

Back at our camp, Nate stepped carefully over his dirt sketch and I made sure to avoid it too.

He pointed to the two circles. "A hundred and sixty-five million years ago, the Earth spun on its axis four hundred times for every one revolution around the Sun. The days were a little shorter back then, but there were thirty-five more of them every year."

"You mean the Earth is spinning slower today?"

"Everything in the universe begins to lose energy from the moment it is born. One day this planet could stop spinning altogether, if it isn't swallowed up by the dying Sun first."

"That's inspiring."

"That's reality. Everything slows down and eventually dies. It's also true that the speed at which something loses energy is usually predetermined, set by the laws of physics. But we humans have been blessed with the unique ability to control the speed of our decline. Using free will, we can accelerate it or slow it down."

Nate untied his pack and laid out his bedroll. I did the same, and we both stretched out on our sleeping bags. I was beginning to get a little chilly in my sweat-damp shirt.

"Remember, the human body is an amalgamation of seventy-five trillion cells."

"Yeah, it's a universe in there."

"Those cells have limited life spans. As they age and become unviable, they divide and pass their DNA on to a new generation of cells. We are mortal because our cells can divide only a finite number of times before they die. That number is predetermined and out of our control. When a cell dies, the tissue it belongs to begins to die. Ultimately, organs and systems fail, and the body dies, too.

"But—and this is important—we humans are capable of controlling how fast our cells age, the rate at which they are forced to divide, and consequently, the length of our lives."

Maybe it was my exhaustion, but I couldn't quite wrap my brain around that idea. "Control how fast our cells age?"

"Let's say the average cell can divide a hundred times. If each of its replacements is viable for only six months, how much time will pass before that cell divides for the last time?"

"Half a year multiplied by a hundred. Fifty years."

"Correct. Now, what if we were able to extend the life span of each generation to, say, twelve months?"

"One year times a hundred, that's a hundred years. You'd double the lifespan."

Nate sat upright and, adopting the tone of a pilgrim seeking spiritual enlightenment, said, "Wise Master, I realize that if I want to live a long and healthy life I must feed my body high-quality food, eat consciously, and stay active. I know that I must fast from time to time to keep its work area clean, and meditate daily to prevent stress from doing it harm. But I sense there is something I have overlooked."

I straightened myself and slapped on a serious expression. "The secret, my ignorant disciple, is to maximize the life span of each new generation of cells."

"And what must I do to achieve such a wondrous outcome?" he asked with mock excitement.

"Hold the phone, supplicant, Swami must consult the celestial spirits."

I closed my eyes and lifted my palms to the sky in a ridiculously grand gesture.

"I have received their response."

"What is it, Wise One?"

"The health and longevity of the body is dependent on the health and longevity of its individual cells…"

"Yes?"

"Sleep, Grasshopper, is the final key—and not when I'm talking. You must get enough sleep to provide your cells the downtime they need for repair and maintenance. That is the key to extending their lives, and yours."

"Thank you, Master." Nate looked confused. "Grasshopper?"

"It's from *Kung Fu*. TV? Never mind."

He raised an eyebrow. "And the downtime, Master, how much sleep do I need?"

I thought for a second. "Take yourself to the mountaintop, Grasshopper. The answer awaits you there."

The two of us cracked up, and by the time we settled down, night was falling fast. It was good to stretch out, even on a sleeping bag on the ground. I felt myself drifting. The next time he spoke, Nate reclaimed the role of teacher.

"In 1879, Thomas Edison perfected the incandescent light bulb. Three years later, he came up with a way to generate enough electricity to light entire cities at night. That year, people began to sleep an hour and a half less than before.

"Ninety minutes may not sound like a lot of time, but it's an entire sleep cycle. With the invention of movies, television, and other forms of nighttime distraction, the situation has only gotten worse. These days, virtually everyone is sleep-deprived."

"So, here we are on a mountaintop, with none of those distractions. Are we at least going to build a fire?" I asked, rubbing my hands together. The temperature was dropping.

Nate removed his shoes. "Too dangerous, the brush here is like kindling."

He slipped into his bedroll and tucked a folded blanket under his head. "Full moon's gonna rise in a little while. That'll be nice."

Then he yawned, turned onto his side and didn't say another word.

I changed into my thermal underwear, climbed inside my sleeping bag and stared into the blackening sky. In awhile, the moon rose and everything on Two Gulls glowed in a soft and silver light.

∞

The chattering of birds woke me. I pulled the sleeping bag over my head against the cold air.

"Good morning, morning glory," Nate said cheerfully. "Yes, it seems you are a morning glory after all. How are you feeling?"

I sat up, making sure to keep the covers around me. "Pretty good, considering."

He stood at the head of his bedroll. Then he took a deep breath, released it and launched into a series of flowing movements I recognized as the hatha yoga sun salutation. He went gracefully from pose to pose, synchronizing his inhalation and exhalation with each change. After repeating the series several times, he motioned to me.

"We're here in the trees, son. Want to see what tree pose feels like in a place like this?"

He stepped easily into the crane-like one-legged position, with his left leg bent, sole pressed into his standing right thigh. I did the same, remembering how cocky I'd been the first time I tried.

"Shall we?" he said, closing his eyes.

Fully prepared to lose my balance, I let my eyelids fall, and to my amazement, they were the only things that did. I felt rooted somehow, like the pines around us. I took a few deep breaths, and when I opened my eyes again, he was there, still on one leg, watching me. He didn't say anything, but I could read his face. It said, "You've come a long way."

"You know how to end the practice, right?" he asked, rolling onto his back, extending his legs and letting them fall open. His arms dropped to his sides and he lay, eyes closed, breathing slowly and deeply. I crawled onto my sleeping bag and rested that way for a minute or two, before sitting up. Finally, he bent his knees and rolled onto his side. "You have any trouble getting to sleep last night?" he asked.

"I was awake long enough to watch the moon rise."

"That's not surprising. It could take you a week or so to readjust to Earth time."

"You don't honestly expect me to be in bed at six o'clock every night, do you?"

He pressed up into a seated position. "We spent the night up here because I wanted you to feel how your body responds to the Earth's rhythm in the absence of artificial light. I'll bet you were asleep by seven thirty."

"It was dark, what else was I going to do?"

"Exactly! The point is, even on the longest day of the year there are nine and a half hours of darkness. On the shortest it's dark for over fourteen. You know anybody that's not narcoleptic who sleeps fourteen hours a day?"

I laughed. "Of course not."

"So—how many hours do you figure you slept last night?"

I checked my watch—it was five forty-five. "About ten hours."

"Ten hours! Are you sure you're not narcoleptic?" He chuckled. "Actually, that sounds about right. If this were June and not the end of October, you probably could've made do with eight. As I said last night, on the whole, folks need between eight and ten hours. But most of 'em barely get seven—and they're the wrong seven at that."

He interlocked his fingers, reached his arms over his head and stretched slowly from side to side.

"There's a big difference between restorative sleep and just plain being unconscious. Generally speaking, the darkest hours of the day are from eight at night to four in the morning. Those are the core restorative hours when your body is calibrated to do its healing.

"So no, I don't expect you to be in bed at six o'clock. But I will say this: Every hour past eight you're doing anything but sleeping is one less hour your body has to keep you young and in good repair."

"Let me get this straight: If I go to bed at midnight and wake up at eight in the morning—"

"You're only getting four hours of restorative sleep—not exactly a recipe for vitality and longevity."

"I hear you, but I've been a night person my entire adult life."

"Yes, you have. And now you're suffering for it."

He lowered his arms.

"I knew this lesson would be a challenge for you. That's why I saved it for last. Let's just see how it goes, okay?"

"You're the boss." I crossed my legs and lay my hands on my thighs, palms up. "Can we meditate, please? All this talk about getting to bed early is stressing me out."

THIRTY-THREE

The truth was, I'd slept well, and I felt especially refreshed as we hiked back through the canyon to Nate's place. The early morning had a quality all its own—calm and clean. There seemed to be an inherent potential and promise at the birth of a new day that made it easy to feel hopeful. And I *was* hopeful. The lessons I'd gotten from Nate were like taking the car apart in the driveway. It felt chaotic, seeing the elements of my life strewn around in new ways. As things came together, though, I began to feel better, and it seemed like I could accomplish anything. Of course, this was a kind of trial run outside the pressures of a job or friends or "real life." But something in the morning air made me think I could manage that too.

"Why don't you wash up," Nate said as we clomped up to his front porch. "I'll make us some breakfast. Then there's something I want to show you."

He pointed to an open doorway on the opposite side of the living room. "Bathroom's through there. I only light the water heater in emergencies and haven't had one of those for years. Anyway, a cold shower's good for the circulation."

Cold shower? Holy hell! If I wasn't covered from head to toe with yesterday's dried sweat and dust, I might have taken a pass. But I'd survived a night out in "the elements" and was feeling, dare I say, rugged.

That lasted until the water hit my chest. Its cold punch knocked the wind out of me and sent my entire central nervous system into shock. I let out a loud yelp.

Nate's laughter carried all the way from the kitchen.

I soaped up, rinsed off and got out of that torture chamber as fast as I could.

Nate cackled through the bathroom door. "Invigorating, isn't it?"

I hated to admit it, but actually, it was. "Yep," I yelled. "I'll have to try that again in twenty or thirty years."

"Suit yourself. Breakfast is on the table."

I dried off, got into fresh clothes and joined him in the dining room. He sat behind a couple of bowls, one with yogurt and fruit and another containing granola, something I hadn't eaten since college. I had vague memories of sweet, sticky-hard nuggets that could've broken your teeth. But with a splash of cold goat's milk, Nate's homemade granola was actually delicious—nutty and not too sweet. The meal was a far cry from my old standby—bagel and coffee—and I was surprised how much I enjoyed it.

I was taking my time, but I noticed Nate was eating a little more quickly than usual, and he seemed eager to get on with the day.

"Just drop those plates in the sink," he said, heading into the living room.

I rinsed and stacked the bowls and dried my hands on the front of my shirt.

"Step lively, boy." There was a distinctly urgent tone in that voice. I half ran through the dining room and stopped short when I saw what Nate was holding.

"What have you got there?" I asked.

"It's a guitar. I thought you played these things."

"I know it's a guitar. What's it doing here?"

"My father gave this to me. He thought it might help me get over my troubles." Nate wrapped his arms around the instrument. "I expect Heather told you that I lost my wife and child."

I nodded and felt a lump rise in my throat.

"Well," he said, "I never did get the hang of this thing—hold on to it for sentimental reasons. Here," he took the guitar by the neck and held it out. "What do you think?"

I had never seen a guitar like this before, except in picture books of vintage acoustic instruments. It was what they used to call a parlor guitar—hourglass shaped and three-quarter sized. I took it from him and held it in front of me. Its tuners were set sideways, as they usually are on classical models, though this was a steel string. A floral pearl inlay decorated the face of the open headstock that sat at the top of its ivory-bound ebony fingerboard. The lacquer on its spruce top had aged to a gorgeous mellow tan. The sides and back were made of Brazilian rosewood, a rare wood with an exceptional tone. Because it came from an endangered tree, it was banned for use in guitar making decades ago, so you hardly ever saw one. Most striking of all, the instrument was in mint condition.

I ran my hand over its smooth curves.

Nate cleared his throat. "You gonna make love to it or play it?"

"No, no. Yes, of course." I sat on the arm of the couch and reached into my pocket for the thumb pick I always carried.

He seemed impressed. "You come prepared."

"I learned a long time ago that you never know when a guitar will appear."

I fingered an E chord and ran the pick across the strings. It was in perfect tune.

"Are these new strings?" I asked.

"Heather plays it pretty regular. She says guitars need playing to maintain their tone."

"She's right," I said. "The vibrations keep the top resonant." I began to finger-pick an old Jimmy Cox blues tune. The guitar's sound was bright and full, with a perfect balance of treble and bass.

Nate's face lit up. "'Nobody Knows You When You're Down and Out'—you know the whole tune?"

"Sure, why?"

"Key of C, right?" he asked, pulling a dark mahogany case off the bookshelf. He set it down on the coffee table and opened the lid. Inside was a set of harmonicas, neatly arranged in individual velvet housings.

"Wait, you play?"

"Don't watch TV, and a man can only read so much." He pulled a harmonica out, cupped it in his hands and blew into it. The sound was strong and bluesy. He bent notes and used his hands to shape the harp's tone as well as the best players I'd ever heard. I launched into the song's introduction: C, E7, A7, D minor, A7, D minor. Then Nate joined in, riffing over the second half: F, D7, C, A7.

The guitar played like a dream.

"You take the verse," he said and blew a descending melody line as the progression worked its way around to the root...D7, G7, C.

I sang:

Once I lived the life of a millionaire
Spent all my money, I just didn't care
Took all my friends out for a good time
Bought boot-leg whiskey, champagne, and wine...

At the chorus, Nate played fills between the vocal lines.

'Cause, nobody knows you
When you're down and out
In your pocket, not one penny
And as for friends, you don't have any...

Nate took the next verse, transitioning into a soaring improvisation over the last four bars. The guy was seriously good—chills-up-your-spine good. When the chorus came around again, I let him keep wailing. Then I joined him to wrap it up:

Nobody knows you
Nobody knows you
Nobody knows you when you're down and out

I gave Nate a big smile. "Whoa, you are a *player*, man!"

"I get by. You're pretty good yourself. So you like the blues?"

"Blues, yeah, some, mostly folk. I'm an old folkie at heart. But there's no money in it these days. House, pop, hip-hop, bubble gum, country, light jazz—that's where the market is, so that's what I write…try to anyway. But whenever I'm at my wits' end, I play a little blues or folk music, and I feel better."

Nate frowned. "What a shame. Seems to me a writer ought to write what's in his heart."

"Not if he wants to eat." That quick, defensive reply shocked me. After all, I knew what I was getting into when I decided to write songs for a living.

There was a long silence. Nate cleared the harmonica with several sharp raps to his thigh and placed it back in its case.

"This is a beautiful instrument," I said, cradling the old guitar.

Nate walked over and stood in front of me. "Play the open strings one at a time."

I struck the low E string, then the A string, the D, G, B, and finally, the high E string.

"Let's say each of those strings represents one of the six aspects of an authentic life, lived in harmony with nature."

He plucked the bottom E.

"Eat food high in Life Force, designed by nature, not man."

Then the top E.

"Eat with a conscious intention to receive the food's gifts. Intention dictates outcome. The best food won't do you any good if it isn't digested and absorbed."

He hit the A string.

"In the spring and autumn, steer clear of food for a few days, to give your digestive system a rest and your body a chance to clean house."

And then the D string.

"Move this body. Live an active life."

Then he brushed the G.

"But take the time to be still. Quiet your mind everyday to give your body a chance to throw off stress and to allow universal wisdom to guide you."

Finally, he ran his thumb across the B string.

"Synchronize your life with the planet's circadian rhythm to get the downtime you need for repair and maintenance. You were born a human being, not a bat."

He strummed all six strings. "Play something else for me."

I started finger picking "Alice's Restaurant," an anti-Establishment song Arlo Guthrie wrote in the late sixties.

"Great tune," he said. "A bit irreverent for his father's taste, I imagine."

"Well, Woody did die the year Arlo released that record."

Nate grimaced. Then he turned his attention to my fingers, intently watching both my hands as I moved through the chord progression.

"Keep playing," he said as he reached out and detuned the B string. Immediately, the sound became jarring and discordant.

I stopped.

"Something wrong?" he asked coyly.

"Yeah, you put the guitar out of tune."

"That's not exactly accurate. Five of those strings are in tune. Only one is out."

"Right, but you know I can't play it this way."

His eyes got wide. "Ah, so, all six strings have to be in tune before you can make music on that guitar." He stroked his chin. "Very interesting."

"Come on, you know that."

"Are you sure you can't make do with three or four?"

I gave him an incredulous look.

He mimicked it and laughed. "Son, this body of yours is a magnificent instrument of nature, capable of making beautiful music too. Your life has the potential to be rich and full, with all the physical, mental, and creative energy you could possibly want." He dropped his hand and sat on the edge of the coffee table. "But lately, that hasn't been your experience, now has it?"

I smirked at him.

"Before you can make beautiful music on *this* instrument," he pointed a finger at me, "what do you have to do?"

"Tune it."

"And how will you do that?"

I felt like a third-grader. "By using the lessons you've taught me."

"How many of those lessons, one, two, three?"

"All of them."

He cupped his ear and cocked his head toward me. "I'm sorry, say again."

"Give me a break, Nate. Okay, all of them. I have to put all six lessons into action."

"You sure you can't make due with three or four?"

"God, you are a pain in the ass. Here, take this," I held out the guitar, "before I get too attached. That's a great ax, man."

He returned it to its hard-shell case. Then he reached into his pocket and pulled out a folded piece of paper. "It's gonna take about eight weeks to build that greenhouse for Heather. I assume I can count on you to see it through to the finish."

"Yes, of course." I figured it was small bill for everything I'd received.

"Good." He unfolded the paper. "I've taken the liberty of putting together a training schedule that I want you to follow until we're done. He handed me the paper and I read:

Monday through Friday:
Rise at dawn.
Meditate for twenty minutes.
Be at the work site within one hour of sunrise.
Eat a light breakfast.
Work on the greenhouse until noon.
Break for lunch.
Back to work until 3:00 p.m.
Wash up.
Hike to Two Gulls.
Meditate for twenty minutes at the summit.
Hike down and go home.
Eat an early dinner.
Get to bed by 8:00 p.m.
Saturday and Sunday:
No work.
Reduce food intake—Fresh vegetable juice for breakfast and dinner, vegetarian lunch.

"Okay." I refolded the paper and slipped it into my shirt pocket. My mind was already racing.

"You can do what you want once we're finished building the greenhouse. But until then, I expect you to follow those instructions to the letter." He grabbed the harmonica case and returned it to the bookshelf. "Now get going. I'm giving you the rest of the day off. We start work tomorrow."

THIRTY-FOUR

Another crossroads. Since childhood, I had been aware of liminal moments, which I usually recognized only later, when I abandoned old habits or beliefs in favor of new ones that permanently altered the course of my life. Some awakenings came with a start, like having to admit to myself—after jumping off the garage roof—that I couldn't fly. Nate was right: accepting the fact of gravity really *is* a big step toward wisdom.

Other new truths were easier on the body, but just as profound. I remember sitting in a pitch meeting one afternoon and realizing with a start that everyone else did *not* have their act together. It was as though a light pinged on: I wasn't the only screwup. I might as well take some chances.

I could go along for years, even decades, in a kind of sameness and then suddenly experience one of these shifts in consciousness and behavior. And every time, the pattern was the same. Invariably, I would feel a fair amount of resistance to the new idea, which had to be overcome. I'd make a little progress, backslide, and somehow find that I wanted to keep going.

This training schedule was a huge threshold to cross, a mother lode of change—as in, taking over my entire life and replacing practically every habit and routine with something new. I couldn't do it quietly on my own, either—it would affect Merry, of course, and our friends too. Getting out to a concert, a movie, or even a dinner party in the evening—all of that would be going away for the next weeks. And if I kept on with it, it was going to be hard to explain to people that, "Oh by the way, I go to bed at eight, just like your kids!"

I'd hated "eccentric" eating enough that I made fun of Merry's vegetarian recipes until she gave up and started cooking us burgers. Now I was Mr. "local and organic." I felt my old friend resistance popping up, but the big question I kept circling back to was: What's the alternative? I'd staggered over to Nate's that first time with no passion and no energy. Was I supposed to go back to that?

I thought a lot about my dumpster episode and the grease of that last burrito as I contemplated the challenges that lay ahead. It was like aversion therapy to remember how I used to feel. And I solidified my resolve to see my training through to the finish by conjuring a hideous outcome as the price of failure: cancer, stroke, diabetes, paralysis, divorce, economic ruin, homelessness, the feeling that the studio was a coffin and the thing I loved most, music, was killing me.

I summoned up that frightening litany repeatedly during the first two weeks of Nate's boot camp. Things got off to a rocky start—literally. Dismantling the stone wall, a boulder at a time, and reconstructing it some thirty feet away felt an awful lot like forced labor, senselessly moving a rock pile from one end of a prison yard to another.

Merry's eyes nearly came out of her head when I showed her the training schedule. She was happy to think differently about the way we ate, and she'd been a meditator when I met her. But in four years of marriage, she rarely saw me get to sleep before eleven or wake before nine. The idea of my getting to bed at eight o'clock seemed ludicrous to both of us. And she was a night owl, too. Thankfully, we had license to disappear from our social life for a couple of months. No one expects new parents to be out late at night.

As it turned out, getting to bed at eight was easy. After hauling rocks for six hours a day, day after day, I could barely keep my eyes open at dinner and often collapsed into bed well before eight. Pretty soon I was waking at dawn without the help of an alarm clock.

But the physical labor was hard on my back, which went into spasm every couple of days. Nate was sympathetic, but that didn't get me off hard time at the rock pile. After treating me five or six times with smelly, hot compresses, he just added sun salutations to our pre-breakfast routine to stretch and strengthen my back muscles and loosen my spine. By the end of the third week, the rock wall was completely relocated, and my back was no longer complaining.

At three each afternoon, Nate handed me a canteen and a small satchel containing fruit and nuts, and pushed me out the front door. I'd lumber across the open field on legs that felt too tired to carry me, then shuffle down into the ravine where I'd find a boulder beside the creek and sit for several minutes before attempting the arduous trek to Two Gulls. A few times I was so worn out, I fell asleep during meditation and came to after sundown, with barely enough time to head back to Nate's before dark.

Once, after arriving inordinately late, I found him playing harmonica on the steps in front of his darkened house.

"Why don't you turn on a few lights?" I asked.

He lowered the harmonica long enough to say, "Got no lights. Don't need 'em."

He was probably the only person in Los Angeles County voluntarily living without electric lighting. And by all appearances, he was better off for it.

As our project took shape, so did my body and new way of life. In a few weeks, I had energy to burn when I woke in the morning—and nothing hurt. The morning routine felt...normal. The work was challenging, but I was careful to pace myself, and before long, I was keeping up with Nate.

On Saturdays, Merry and I took the baby to Maggie G's market to shop for fresh produce and stock up on vegetable juice for the weekends. My new diet was simple—vegetables and fruit, raw nuts and seeds, poultry and fish, whole grains, and of course, goat yogurt, courtesy of Gracie. I ate no processed or refined food, nothing out of a box or can, and I didn't even think about the sugary and starchy foods that were staples of my old diet.

By mid-November, I managed to clear the brush, turn the soil, and remove the largest rocks from the three-hundred-square-foot area that Nate had marked with string. Our lessons completed, there were no more lectures, no more metaphorical stories. In fact, we talked very little at all, and I started to wonder if he was distancing himself in preparation for my departure.

He surprised me one morning by asking, "You got plans for Thanksgiving? Heather's coming over and we'd like you and your family to join us—if you're free."

We were. Merry's parents had passed away years before, and my mother and adoptive father were divorced and living far away. The two couples who'd become part of our own Thanksgiving tradition—Geoffrey and his ex-wife Bobbi, whom I'd known since college, and their respective partners—had other plans this year. Merry was relieved not to have to organize anything, and I was glad I wouldn't have to face down a huge buffet in some restaurant.

The old man and I worked right up to the holiday, leveling the ground, digging a foot-deep trench around the entire perimeter and installing wooden forms at the bottom for the concrete footing.

On the Tuesday of Thanksgiving week, I got home to find Geoffrey and a girl young enough to be his daughter entwined on our living room couch. We hadn't seen each other since the day he'd sent me to "rehab," and since we wouldn't be carving a turkey together this year, he wanted to see how I was doing.

Over dinner, we learned that he and the girl met at a recording studio where she's the receptionist. Geoffrey had become the new "Barbie King," producing all the music for Mattel's current ad campaign, and he was working on national spots for Pabst Blue Ribbon beer and Sprint.

Before leaving, he pulled me aside for a word in private. "Let me know if things get tight, okay? You could produce a couple of Pabst spots for me." I told him I'd think about it and get back to him. It's odd, he was making money hand-over-fist writing jingles, and I was hauling rocks. But, aside from the money part, it felt like I had the better deal.

"So, what do you think?" I said to Merry after they'd left. "Can you see your husband in the jingle business?"

"Not if it's going to do to you what it's doing to him."

"What do you mean?"

"Did you see what he looked like? Death warmed over. He seemed so stressed —that clenching and unclenching thing he was doing with his jaw. Did he ever stop jiggling his leg? And he's so pale." She laughed. "It's not really funny, but I kept thinking during dinner that the two of you looked like the before and after pictures of some miracle health system." She put down the dishes she was holding and gave me a hug. "If you had to give up what you've accomplished in the last couple of months to have what he's got, I'd say it's not worth it."

At Nate's the next morning, he and a man named Carl were unhitching a gasoline-powered cement mixer from a pickup truck loaded with sand, gravel, and bags of cement. Carl, a contractor and one of Nate's former students, had donated the mixer and concrete ingredients and was going to help us pour the foundation.

He handed me goggles and gloves and put me in charge of filling buckets with sand and gravel, which he combined with cement and water in the mixer. Getting the consistency just right required an expertise that Nate and I lacked, and we were content to handle the grunt work of transferring the finished batches into wheelbarrows, carting them to the trench and pouring the mixture into the wooden forms. It was work all right, but what a vacation compared to hauling rocks! I smiled to think of how hard it had been for me to push the much lighter wheelbarrows of compost only a couple of months before.

The three of us spent most of the day on the project, with Carl doing the finish work, smoothing and leveling the surface with a trowel.

As we wound down, Heather stopped by to go over the blueprints with Nate. I took the excuse to rest and thought I'd join their conversation. But the technical language—photosynthetic capacity, wind load, isolated solar gain—was way over my head, so I decided to make myself useful and hauled the last pile of cleared brush down to the compost bins.

On her way out, Heather gave me a hug. "What do you say we bring our guitars tomorrow and make some music?"

"Sure," I said. I hadn't played in weeks.

We pulled up in the Volvo on Thanksgiving Day with a sweet potato pie and green bean casserole that Merry made for the feast. She carried the food, and I took Zoë up to the porch in her baby carrier. The smell of roasted turkey and baked apples filled the house.

Merry and Nate embraced and gave each other a look that I took for mutual gratitude and affection. Zoë landed in everyone's arms—but she remained the longest in Nate's. The two of them seemed perfectly content together as we sat in the living room while the ladies set the table.

"She's a beauty, so full of life," he said, looking down at the baby. He smiled, stroking her fine hair as she rested against him. "It took me a long time to get over losing my wife and our baby," he said quietly.

"The pain must have been terrible."

He looked up at me. "Something tells me that you know what it feels like to lose someone."

"My biological father abandoned our family when I was very young."

He cradled Zoë and looked into her sweet face. "It's hard to imagine how someone could walk away from their own child."

"Yeah, well…" I could feel myself shutting down, the way I always did when emotions came too close.

Nate rose, brought Zoë to me and laid her in my arms. "I realized a long time ago that if I was ever going to open my heart again, I had to get past that pain. Otherwise, the bastards win again." He mussed my hair. "Don't let the bastard win."

Nate headed for the kitchen to put the bird on a platter, and after Merry nursed Zoë and put her down in the bedroom for a nap, the four of us joined hands at the holiday table. Heather offered a short prayer for "peace, international cooperation, and man's awakening to the truth about himself." Nate thanked nature for her delicious gifts and asked everyone to "remain mindful of the life-sustaining benefits this food offers our bodies." Merry and I added hearty amens.

As we ate, I was surprised to see the way Nate drew Merry out. We'd so often chewed together in silence that I wasn't used to this more social side of him. "What line of work are you in?" he asked her.

"I'm an executive assistant at an entertainment law firm—or will be when my maternity leave ends."

"And what did you do before that?"

"For about fifteen years, I sang and danced on tour with Olivia Newton-John, Loretta Lynn, and Mac Davis."

"A performer, how exciting. Do you miss it? How is it being a new mother?"

This went on for awhile, but when Merry turned the questions on him, Nate spoke only about the garden and the orchard. He never mentioned the work he and I were doing together, never asked her how she felt about the changes I was making. He never even mentioned the lessons or the precarious state of the world he cared so much about. That information, it appeared, was for students who'd sought him out. He wasn't, as I'd feared in the early days, a zealot without an off switch.

After dinner, Heather and I did the dishes while Nate gave Merry a tour of the garden. When we regrouped in the living room for tea and baked apples, Heather went straight for her guitar. "I hear you like folk music," she said.

I pulled my guitar from its case and for the next couple of hours the two of us led our little group through some of the greatest folk songs ever written—tunes by Bob Dylan, Pete Seeger, Woody Guthrie, Phil Ochs, Gordon Lightfoot, Paul Simon, Tom Paxton, and, of course, Joni Mitchell—protest songs whose political and social messages still moved us. We all joined in, working out the harmonies as we went along. Nate took the instrumental breaks, and his harmonica added a rich texture to our sound.

After a heartfelt rendition of "If I Had a Hammer," I told the story of seeing Peter, Paul and Mary play at my college in the late sixties. I met Mary Travers when I went backstage after their second show to take her a corned beef sandwich. She'd announced during their first set that she couldn't find a good one in our little town, and I'd gone out to prove her wrong. She was so taken with my gesture that she invited me to walk her back to her room at the student union, where we talked and she read me poetry that became lyrics on their next album.

Heather seemed awestruck by the story and lamented being born too late to take part in the folk movement. That got me thinking about my own musical journey. I'd been a folkie for years before it went out of fashion. And nothing I had done professionally in the last two decades brought me as much joy. Playing folk music felt like coming home. I wanted to make music—*this* kind of music. And if there was no money in it, well, that was a wrinkle I'd have to iron out. Somehow, the joy was all that seemed to matter.

Folk was simple, honest—words that fit Nate too. His life was so different from mine—uncomplicated, unhurried, and unaffected by the whims of a capricious professional world. He planted something, tended it, and it grew. The allure of that kind of life—the one I'd been immersed in for the past six weeks—was extraordinary. Not that I could ever be a farmer. But I could find something real to do. Nate had been an engineer and he'd found a way.

As we sang, I felt the depth of his gift to me. No matter where I chose to go from here, I'd have the health and energy to get me there. And on this day of thanksgiving, I was overcome with gratitude.

༄

Construction on the greenhouse went into full swing that Friday. First, we built the wall forms and poured the concrete.

Then Carl brought in another set of skilled hands to help us assemble the aluminum frame and construct the back and side walls. I was everyone's assistant, helping to install doors, vents, gutters, and downspouts. The real transformation came when the south wall glazing went up, two sparkling layers of glass, embedded in putty, spaced six inches apart, and set precisely at a 44-degree angle to the horizon to capture maximum sunlight.

When the work moved inside, Heather stopped by now and then to check our progress and go over some of the finer considerations specific to orchid cultivation—ventilation, air flow, humidity, and temperature control.

We spent the week before Christmas building the greenhouse's upper and lower benches, painting the concrete walls, and laying the gravel floor. Finally, we rolled in six 55-gallon drums, set them against the back wall and filled them with water. Their purpose, I was told, was to absorb the sun's heat to keep the greenhouse a tropical, orchid-friendly temperature at night.

By mid-December, our work was nearly complete, and my training seemed to be reaching its final stages. I knew it in my body as I hiked to Two Gulls, a ritual that had long since ceased to feel like punishment. My legs and lungs could easily transport me through the ravine and up to the mountain's summit, and now I could enjoy the scenery.

The chatter in my head gradually quieted too, and my meditations became deep and restful. For the first time in my life, I found that I could be profoundly relaxed yet extraordinarily alert. Often during meditations, melodies or ideas for songs would float into my mind, and I began bringing pencil and paper with me to jot them down. But I'd lost my compulsion to turn my inspirations into anything commercial. Maybe I'd show them to Geoffrey someday...maybe not. I could feel my musical soul again, and I wasn't about to risk losing it.

Best of all, Nate had become family. Nearly every Sunday, I took Merry and Zoë to visit with him, and Heather would often join us for a vegetarian potluck brunch where we'd play and sing folksongs for hours.

The fear and desperation I'd felt my entire career was gone, replaced with a sense of hope.

THIRTY-FIVE

Finishing the greenhouse the day before Christmas was no coincidence. The project was a gift to all of us. Nate finally had a proper place to start seedlings for the garden. Heather would be able to get her orchid business going to save for college. And I had proof that I could do something besides make music. I could look at our work and see something tangible and permanent that I'd helped to build with my own two hands. I could handle a physical challenge; I knew that now. And, Jesus, I had stuck to that insane training schedule and come out the other side a different person. My pains and bloated belly were gone. My energy was back. I was strong, and I could actually say I felt youthful. Those gifts, all of them, were priceless.

༄

Merry was restless a couple of days after the holiday and wanted to take Zoë for a walk on the Santa Monica Pier.

She'd been cooped up in the house, entertaining family and friends, and seemed a bit weary from fielding all their questions about my "midlife crisis" and this strange new lifestyle I'd immersed myself in.

"When I tell people what you've been doing they act as if you've gone off the deep end," she told me with a smile. "But I just tell them how happy I am for you, how good this is."

I bent to the couch where she was sitting with Zoë and gave her a quick kiss.

"Okay if I run up to see Nate? I can swing by for you and the baby on my way back."

"Be sure to tell him I miss him and we'll come up soon." she said.

Since Nate and I had finished our work there was no real reason to call on him. But I had a vague sense of threads left hanging, and it was gnawing at me.

When I walked up, he and another man were sitting in the porch rockers, engaged in a lively discussion. Nate saw me and held up a hand to pause their conversation.

"Sam!" he called. "Glad you stopped by. There's someone here I want you to meet."

The two men rose as I joined them.

"Sam, this is my good friend Al. Al, this is Sam. He's just finished his training."

Al was a tall, good-looking man about my age. He smiled warmly. "Congratulations," he said, giving my hand a firm shake, "and welcome to the club." Then, in a pleasant, resonant voice that had a hint of a Southern drawl he added, "What are you going to do with the knowledge you've just received?"

Nate laughed. "Easy, Al. Sam's still digesting all this. He's gonna need some time to figure that out."

Al sat back into his chair with a look of mild disappointment.

Nate remained standing. "Al's a United States senator—being direct is an occupational hazard. You'll find he doesn't mince words."

I caught Al's eye. "Well," I said, "that's a quality I admire. I'm sure you know this old guy has a tendency to cut to the chase too."

"Touché." Nate chuckled and stepped off the porch. "Gentlemen, if you'll excuse me, I want to see how Heather's coming along in the greenhouse. You should get to know each other."

Nate disappeared around the corner of the house.

"So, Al, what brings you to California?" I lowered myself into Nate's empty seat.

"I wanted to get his feedback on a book I'm writing," he replied.

"What's the book about?"

"Our ecological predicament. The scientific evidence is compelling, but often technical. I translate it into plain English, offer some remedies and call on governments and individuals to take responsibility for this planet."

"Sounds terrific. What's it called?"

"No title yet. I thought maybe Nate could help with that."

He leaned back in the rocker. "So, what line of work are you in?"

"Music business, but I'm thinking about trying something else—not sure what."

Al looked thoughtful. "Maybe you'll find a way to spread the word, be a part of the solution."

I shifted uncomfortably. "This stuff, Nate's lessons...the effects have been great, really amazing. It's just..."

"What?"

"The whole notion of an endangered, invisible biofield— is so incredible."

Al took a deep breath. "Uh-huh. Do you believe it exists?"

"I haven't seen it, have you?"

"I'm not sure, maybe. From what I understand, not everyone is able to. But I *am* sure that this world is in deep, man-made trouble." He paused. "Have you got kids?"

"A baby girl, seven months old."

"I have four, myself. Almost lost my boy in an accident a couple of years ago. Let me tell you, Sam. Something like that puts things into perspective pretty quick." He grabbed the arms of the chair and rocked forward. "Preserving the environment was a key political issue for me long before I studied with Nate. My wife and I have a mutual love for nature, and we've always used our vacations to escape the city to show our kids what's real, help them understand what really matters.

"But since the accident, I'm absolutely certain that nothing I do with my life is as important as protecting this planet for my children and their children." He locked eyes with me. "If you care about the kind of world you're going to leave your daughter, you can't afford to wait for hard evidence that the biofield exists before getting off your ass."

His bluntness took me aback.

"No question this is important," I said. "The entire human population needs to be taught what we know, and then every last person needs to make a wholesale change in their behavior. Otherwise, we're all doomed. It's easy for you to say we should do something about the situation. You've got influence. But who am I? I'm just a regular person. Who's going to listen to me?"

Al threw up his hands. "Oh, so *that's* it. You're just one person, and one person can't make a difference."

"I don't see how, not on that kind of scale."

"Thank God everyone doesn't think like you or nobody in this country would cast a vote."

The two of us sat back to cool down in silence. Finally, Al spoke.

"Have you read the book *Lifetide* by Dr. Lyall Watson?"

"No."

"Ever heard the story of '*The Hundredth Monkey*'?"

"Sorry, I haven't."

"Dr. Watson is an anthropologist, biologist, botanist, ethnologist, zoologist, and author. He's a member of that rare breed of scientists willing to consider the existence of forces and elements that lie beyond the scope of quantitative measurement. In other words, he's a free thinker.

"'*The Hundredth Monkey*' appears in his book, *Lifetide*. Since its publication in 1979, the story has made quite a stir in the scientific community. A few of the statements of the researchers involved were made off the record, which has led many of his peers to label his findings pseudoscience. But I believe he reveals a powerful truth about the nature of consciousness, which is germane to our discussion."

"What's the story?"

"In 1952, on the island of Koshima, a group of primatologists were observing the behavior of the Macaca fuscata, a species of Japanese monkey. The scientists were feeding the monkeys sweet potatoes dropped in the sand.

275

Although the monkeys enjoyed the potatoes, they didn't like the sand.

"One day, a young female solved the problem by washing her sweet potato in a stream. She taught the trick to her mother and playmates, and over the next six years, the scientists witnessed more and more monkeys adopting the habit. But only the adults imitating their children learned to do it—the vast majority of the monkeys on the island, some ten thousand of them, continued to eat the sandy potatoes.

"On an autumn morning in 1958, another monkey, the hundredth monkey, was converted, and by that evening, nearly every monkey on the island was washing potatoes before eating them. What's more amazing, the habit seemed to jump natural boundaries as colonies of monkeys on neighboring islands adopted the behavior.

"Watson theorized that with the addition of the hundredth monkey, the field of awareness associated with the knowledge to wash potatoes reached a critical mass, resulting in an ideological change across an entire population."

Al unfolded the sleeves of his denim shirt and buttoned the cuffs.

"Who will be the 'hundredth monkey' to learn what *you* know?"

He rose from his chair. "You've got more influence than you can possibly imagine," he said softly. "Think what will happen when the knowledge you possess reaches critical mass and everyone in this city begins to live an authentic life in harmony with nature. Then think of another city, and another joining in as this knowledge sweeps across the country and the entire population wakes up to the truth. Can you feel the planet beginning to heal? Don't worry about changing the world. Change your life, share what you've learned and trust that the larger change will happen."

I stood, and we were shaking hands when Nate reappeared. "Al, you ready to go? Al's agreed to help me run a few errands before he heads back to Washington." He stepped between us and threw his arm over my shoulder. "Come back soon, Sam. Be sure you say hello to Heather before you leave."

We exchanged good-byes and the two men walked across the clearing.

"About the title of your book," I heard Nate say as they disappeared into the brush, "try playing with the words 'Earth' and 'balance' and see what you come up with."

THIRTY-SIX

It was warm and sunny at Nate's, but a cold fog had moved in off the ocean by the time Merry and the baby and I arrived at the pier. We drove under the iconic neon sign that had become a potent symbol of the California Dream:

Santa Monica Yacht Harbor
Sport Fishing - Boating
Cafés

The yacht harbor vanished in the late fifties, and the only fishermen on the pier these days looked like poor immigrants trying to catch a cheap meal. But the sign's inaccuracy didn't seem to bother anyone, least of all the hundreds of thousands of tourists who flocked to this place every year to have their pictures taken under it.

I steered the Volvo across the narrow bridge that arced over the roadway below, then down a long concrete ramp and onto the heavy beams of the pier. We passed the old Hippodrome building that housed an ornate, hand-painted carousel, the hundreds of lights over its horses and chariots piercing the mist. I drove slowly past the Crown and Anchor and Boathouse restaurants and turned left at the Playland Arcade into a large open area that had been converted into a parking lot after the Lamonica Ballroom was torn down. It was said that from the shore, the monumental building had appeared to float magically over the water.

On most weekends, the pier is mobbed with visitors. But on this Saturday it was nearly deserted. I figured it was because most people living in Southern California are from someplace else, and during the holidays they all go back there. Whatever the reason, I was glad that Merry and I would have the place pretty much to ourselves.

I stepped from the car into the cold, heavy air.

"Not exactly beach weather," I said.

But Merry was smiling. She's a third-generation Santa Monican, and the pier held countless memories for her. We tucked Zoë into her stroller under a few extra blankets and headed toward the far end, which was barely visible now. A handful of vendors hawked their wares behind makeshift stalls. But farther out, the only sound came from the rhythm of the rolling ocean and the crashing of waves into the pylons beneath us.

The Bait-Tackle Shop, also known as The Last Stop Shop on Route 66, stood at the end of the pier, no more than thirty feet from the iron railing that kept people from falling into the ocean. Officially, the old Interstate terminated at the corner of Lincoln and Olympic, several blocks east. But the way I heard it, sometime in the mid-1930s, someone posted an unofficial sign along Ocean Avenue, just north of the pier that said:

Route 66—End of the Trail

During the Great Depression, the route was brand new, an asphalt ribbon of hope connecting Chicago and the gray, industrialized Midwest to the citrus blooms and beaches of Southern California. It was the Mother Road of Steinbeck's *The Grapes of Wrath* that carried dust bowl migrants to the Promised Land, the Pacific. In people's minds, Route 66 was the road to opportunity, literally.

On the wall outside the entrance to the Bait-Tackle Shop, a giant road map of the United States highlighted the path of the old road. I stopped and traced the southwestern sweep of the decommissioned highway—once indispensable, now a postscript.

"Sam, are you coming?" Merry asked. "We're almost there."

"You go on. I'll catch up."

Over the map the words, 'The End—2,448 Miles,' were printed in bold letters.

The end of the trail. It sure is…for you and me both, old road.

I could still remember stepping onto the stage at a folk club back in Chicago, stumbling into my calling. Chasing that dream brought me here two decades ago. I'd been running ever since, and now, at last, I could stop. No need, anymore, to prove myself or try to impress the father I'd never known.

I pulled my jacket around me against the chill and whispered a prayer into the mist. "What now? Where do I go from here?"

I heard Merry laughing just then, and followed the sound around to the back of the building. She stood at a vendor's stand that faced the end of the pier, having a conversation with someone I couldn't see.

"Sam," she called. "Hungry?"

I checked the carved wooden sign above the stand. It read:

Noah's Ark and Grill

"It's the oddest thing," she said. "I had a sudden taste for my mother's vegetable soup, and the second I thought of it, I noticed the most delicious aroma coming from right here." She sniffed the air. "That smell—just like I remember."

I stepped up to the counter and stretched across to get a good look inside. "Who were you talking to?"

The question brought her back from someplace far away. "I don't know, he must have left for a second."

"Merry, exactly what happened when you found this place? Was a vendor here?"

"No, but the card said to ring the bell for service. So I rang the bell, and...Honey, what's the matter?"

"I'm just curious. So what happened after you rang the bell?"

"Let's see...Zoë distracted me for a second and when I looked back, this nice gentleman was standing there."

I turned and saw Noah, in a white caftan, on the other side of the counter. His eyes were fixed on Merry. "Where were we?" he asked, ladling something steamy into a wooden bowl. "Ah yes, you were telling me about the wonderful soup your mother used to make."

"We grew the vegetables and herbs in our own garden."

"Is that so?"

Merry closed her eyes and inhaled the aroma. "This smells so much like it, really brings me back."

Noah's face beamed. He placed a spoon in the bowl and handed it over the counter to her. "Enjoy," he said, "I hope it brings you many good memories."

They smiled at each other. "Pay the man, would you, honey?" she said. "And get some for yourself. This looks like dinner." She carried the soup in one hand and pushed the stroller with the other to an empty table by the railing.

Noah turned his attention to me. "It's such a shame," he said.

"Oh, you *did* see me. What, what's a shame?"

"We know our Selves so well when we first arrive. But we quickly forget and spend the rest of our lives trying to remember who we really are."

Noah's energy was radiant. He almost glowed.

"Who *are* you?"

"Just a fellow astronaut along for the ride," he said with a laugh.

I stared.

"When I was a kid, I was poor in just about every way possible," he said softly. "But I had an abundance of one thing: intuition. Somehow I could see the truth about people. Didn't have to try, it came natural. Anyway, my family had no money for rent, let alone groceries. I got sick with asthma—nearly died of it. Then one day, a mutual friend of ours rescued me."

"So you *do* know Nate!"

"I was his first student. I thought the lessons seemed crazy at first. But I was desperate, so I learned and applied every one."

His eyes began to shine. "Those lessons saved my life. After my body healed, that gift of mine became more powerful. All I'd have to do is get next to somebody and I could see their pure essence, the child in them, aching to be set free. I worked at it, and pretty soon I could reflect that vision back to people, show them the child safeguarding their true nature. Now and then that glimpse is enough to inspire someone to find their way back." He removed the lid from a pot and gave its contents a stir. "Incidentally, you have a beautiful daughter. Pay attention to her. She's got a lot to teach you."

I looked over at Merry, then back at Noah.

"Don't worry about your wife. She doesn't have as far to travel as you did."

I was sure he was right. "Say, Noah, you wouldn't happen to have a crystal ball back there, would you? I could sure use some help figuring out my next step."

"Don't look at me. I don't have the answer."

"That's too bad. I'd pay good money for it."

"Well, that information isn't for sale. Besides, no one knows the answer but you."

"I know the answer?"

"Always have. You just have to ask yourself the right question."

"Ask myself?"

"Ask. Your. Self."

He filled another soup bowl and set it on the counter. "The beautiful thing about the journey of life, my friend, is that when one trail ends, another begins. That'll be four dollars."

I gave him a five and joined Merry at the table. She seemed far away, lost in thought. So I finished eating and watched the fog move over the water, wondering what the right question might be.

As the light began to fade I heard Noah say, "Do me a favor, Sam. When you're ready to leave, put the bowls on the counter."

"Sure, no problem," I said.

Merry looked up. "What's no problem?"

"It's not a problem for me to take the bowls back to the counter."

"Thanks, honey, I appreciate you handling things without my having to ask."

"I'd love to take credit for the idea, but it was Noah's."

She seemed confused. "What?"

"Just a second ago—didn't you hear?"

When I turned around, Noah was gone. The Ark and Grill was closed and shuttered.

"Never mind," I said.

THIRTY-SEVEN

The sun rose New Year's morning on a day that was going to make Rose Parade organizers ecstatic and the Snow Belt audience envious as hell. Merry was still asleep, so I eased out of bed and into an armchair to meditate.

Ever since Noah suggested having a chat with my Self, meditation had taken on an agenda that made it pretty hard to actually meditate. So, I resolved that morning to let go of any expectations. As Nate said the first time I attempted the climb to Two Gulls: you get there when you get there.

My meditation was deep. Not a single stray thought flitted through my mind. Then I slipped in and out of the shower, and Merry woke as I finished dressing. It was still early—we had both fallen asleep long before midnight.

Traditionally, we observed the passing of one year into the next by sleeping in and watching a rebroadcast of the parade in our bathrobes until noon. French toast, drenched in maple syrup, and an extra cup of coffee or two were usually involved.

Merry and I had been together for six years, and next to my lifestyle, hers always seemed so much healthier. But she had two weaknesses: sugar and caffeine. If I had to guess, I'd say she was addicted to both of them. I hated the idea of encouraging that, but any decision to give up the stuff was hers, not mine. Change for the better is like writing a great tune—you can't force it. People change when they're ready and not before. I was living proof of that.

I made her comfortable on the couch and turned on a live telecast of the parade.

"Sam's Diner is open for business," I said. "What'll it be, lady?"

"The usual, please," she said, glancing between a magazine and the television as the Blue Angels, in tight formation, buzzed Colorado Boulevard and the parade got under way.

I made French toast and coffee for her, fruit and green tea for me, and set the plates on a tray in the middle of the coffee table. It was like a gourmet version of Nate's little test: the apple or the picture-perfect French toast? Merry's breakfast looked and smelled delicious. But I knew exactly how I'd feel if I ate it—first the jitters, then the blood-sugar crash. It was no contest. I grabbed a wedge of apple.

Merry sipped the coffee, set the plate of French toast on her lap and took a bite. "Mmmm, that's so good." She looked at me and the fruit in my hand. "You should know; I don't feel the least bit guilty eating this. It's a special occasion."

"I didn't say anything." I chewed slowly, Nate style.

"You really are going to do this, aren't you?" she said, swirling a bite of the battered bread in syrup.

"I have no intention of being perfect. But, yeah, I'm gonna do the best I can."

"'Cause, you and I don't live on a mountain…we have to live in *this* world."

I knew the idea of giving up sweets and coffee was freaking her out.

"You're right, honey, we do. But Nate proved to me that I have a choice about *how* I want to live in it. And those choices really have a big impact on me and my world. I'm not gonna ask you to do anything you don't want to do. But I can't make believe that I don't know what I know."

She took another long sip of coffee, lingering over it. "Sam," she said, "I think I need to know a little more about what you know—I mean, I see the food part, but there's more to it, right?"

"It's a crazy, idealistic thing, Mer. I think you'll like it," I said. She looked like something out of a photo spread with her softly tangled hair and her breakfast arranged in front of her.

"Okay…"

"I can go into more details later, but here it is in a nutshell: all these little things add up. We eat locally grown food, and a truck isn't spewing exhaust over half the country to get it to us. We go to bed early and the electricity we save reduces the greenhouse gasses belching from a coal-fired power plant. We eat organically grown produce and there are fewer pesticides and chemicals sprayed around. We try to live simply, not waste so much, and there's less garbage out there." The words tumbled out in a rush and I paused for breath. "But here's the thing. If we do it, and our friends do it, and more and more people do it, we can actually heal the planet." I wanted to mention the hundredth monkey, but that could wait.

"You're not kidding, are you," she said, playing with her French toast. "It all sounds so hopeful. *You* sound so hopeful." She raised her fork in a kind of salute. "Happy New Year, honey, I think we're in for something good."

I slid over and gave her a kiss. "Mmmm. Sugar lips."

She set her plate back on the coffee table. "All right," she sighed. "Just shut up and pass the fruit."

We both laughed.

Merry would be going back to work the next day, and in the hours between now and then, she was determined to do as little as possible. When we'd had our fill of parade floats and marching bands, she settled in with her pile of magazines, and I read the paper.

At some point, it dawned on me that in less than twenty-four hours I would be a stay-at-home dad, no longer free to do as I pleased—not that the last few months had felt like a vacation. I had no illusions about how much went into taking care of Zoë, who was crawling now, and I would've been glad to trade places with my wife.

I took charge of changing and feeding the baby when she woke, hoping to put Merry's mind at ease about leaving us to fend for ourselves. But as we played with Zoë that morning, I could see how hard it was going to be for her to spend time away. She didn't want to work, and I felt terribly guilty that she needed to.

The longer I sat on that couch the more restless I became.

"You haven't been up to Nate's for awhile," Merry said. "Why don't you go over and wish him a Happy New Year."

"Maybe." I had purposely put some distance between us to allow space for whatever was supposed to happen next.

"I think you should go." This time it sounded more like a directive. "And give him my love."

∽

Between our house and the Topanga Canyon exit on PCH, I could count the number of cars I passed on one hand. No holiday, save Christmas, has as quieting an effect on the city as New Year's. It's as if the world is in a state of suspended animation. I wondered if the tradition of making New Year's resolutions was connected to the fact that on this day, one of the quietest of the year, people could actually hear themselves think. The Volvo and I sailed to the top of Topanga without encountering another living soul.

As I stepped into the brush and climbed the hill to Nate's, I remembered how frightened and weak I'd felt my first time here—not exactly ready to take the world by storm.

I felt ready now, though—clear-headed and fit. What I lacked, since deciding to take my leave of absence from the music business, was a place to channel all that great energy. What *was* I going to do with the rest of my life?

Halfway across the clearing, I saw Heather coming around the side of the house. "Happy New Year," she said, giving me a big hug. I could sense that something was off.

"Is everything all right? Where's Nate?"

"He's gone."

"What do you mean, 'gone'?"

"He left early this morning for Carmel."

I felt a wave of relief. "Thank God, I thought you meant…"

"Oh no, he's fine…It's his father."

His father! "His father's still alive?"

"Yeah, amazing, isn't it? He's been living on a piece of property he bought in Monterey County over forty years ago, very near the Carmel Mission. But he's slowing down and can't be on his own anymore."

"He's slowing down? How old is the man?"

"Let's see, I think he's about a hundred and ten. Anyway, Nate doesn't think he's got much more time."

"You've got to be kidding me."

Heather grinned. "You sound surprised."

"Well yeah, who lives that long?"

She took my arm and steered me toward the porch. "Nate must have mentioned that longevity was one of the perks of living an authentic life."

"He mentioned something about it. But I didn't take him *that* seriously."

"Well, there you go. How old do you think *he* is?"

"He worked for Hughes during the war? I always thought late sixties, early seventies."

"Ha! Eighty-five!"

I pulled up short. "No way!"

"Way. Nate says people have a choice—they can try to squeeze more life into their days or get more days out of their lives."

"Well, I want to live an authentic life, and I think Merry will too. But let's face it, living that way requires making fundamental changes that don't square with most people's priorities."

Heather's face flushed. "And most people have their heads so far up their asses they can't see what's right in front of them."

"Hey! I'm on your side, remember?"

"Sam," she said, "if you want to be on my side, stop focusing on why this can't work. We're in a battle for our lives and we're badly outnumbered. We need you. If you really want to be on our side, get off the fence."

I could feel my cheeks flush. "Right, right. I'm sorry. It's just—my whole life I thought I knew what mattered. Now everything's upside-down, and I don't know where I fit anymore."

"Don't worry. You'll figure it out." She led me up the porch steps. "Come inside. Nate left you a few things."

Lying on the dining table were two envelopes. She handed me one. I opened it and read:

Invoice for Lessons
Teach someone
Write something

"That's a fair price, don't you think?" she said, handing me the other one.

"Oh yeah. I'll definitely pass along what I've learned."

"Good." She stepped into the living room. "I'll be right back."

I broke the seal on the second envelope and pulled out a single sheet of paper. It was a letter from Nate.

Dear Sam,

I realize how challenging the training was for you, and hope you feel your persistence has paid off—I do. You should be proud of what you have achieved—I am.

Son, you have traveled a long way in a very short time. You stand in new territory at an unfamiliar crossroads and may be wondering which way to turn.

At times like this, I have found that the best way to see forward is to get to higher ground. Get your self to higher ground. I'll be waiting for you.

Nate

PS. The Washburn guitar is yours now. Take good care of her.

I lowered the page as Heather stepped into the room. She was holding Nate's guitar case. "You lucky dog," she said. "Promise you'll let me play it."

"Anytime." I carefully removed the guitar and the two of us admired it for a minute. Then I put it away. "Will you be staying here while Nate's gone?"

"Yeah, I'm going to take care of things till he gets back."

"You need any help?"

"Thanks, I'll be fine. How about you—you need anything?"

I gave her a warm smile. "It's a beautiful day. I was thinking about heading up to Two Gulls. You want to come along?"

"No, you go. I've got work to do. Grab a canteen. And there's some trail mix in the cupboard. I'll see you when you get back." She ran her hand across the top of the guitar case. "You lucky dog!"

∽

I headed to the north side of the property, through the brush and across the meadow. Off in the distance, George and Gracie browsed in the long grass.

I paused a moment where the trail turned down into the canyon that lay between me and Two Gulls and remembered how painful and awkward my first trip this way had been. Not this time. I raced through the switchbacks, sprang across the rocks in the creek, and reached the top of the mountain with energy to spare.

I stopped at the faint drawing of the Sun and Earth that Nate had scratched in the dirt and replayed my dream of the tiny blue dot in space. Could there be a better reason to get up every morning than saving this fragile world? But what exactly could I do?

I hiked farther up to the rock outcropping on the west-facing side of the mountain and took in the view—the long sweep of Topanga Canyon carving its way to the ocean, Nate's place with its garden and orchard and beautiful new green-house, Catalina Island off the coast to the south, Malibu to the north, and the barely perceptible curvature of the Earth where the ocean met the sky.

I felt a strong urge to climb even higher and noticed some footholds in the rock face behind me. Carefully, I scaled the remaining ten feet to the very top.

There, resting in the shallow curve of a wide stone were Nate's pocketknife and a long, freshly cut twig. I picked them up and sat down on the stone's smooth surface. Its contour was a perfect seat.

Without another thought, I began to whittle the twig. As the knife's sharp blade slid under the bark, I remembered the twig Nate had given me in the garden the day we talked about creat-ing a clear vision, how perfectly smooth the wood felt after he removed its rough edges. I wanted my twig to be that smooth, and I wanted to see things as simply and clearly as Nate did. Maybe, if I whittled carefully enough, everything extraneous would fall away and I would know what to do with the rest of my life. The idea should have seemed absurd—but somehow it didn't.

I set my full attention on smoothing that twig. And when I finished, I set the knife down, lay the twig across my open palms, closed my eyes and turned my focus inward.

A breeze caressed my face.

"How can I be of service?" a voice that sounded like mine whispered from deep inside me.

"Just do what you can. That's all," a familiar voice replied.

"Nate?"

"Yes, son."

"I'm so glad. I haven't had a chance to thank you."

"It was my privilege to do what I could do. And now you're ready to go out in the world and do the same."

"But, how?"

"Sam, think about the enlightened people you've met on this journey—Maggie, Heather, Noah, Al, me—different in so many ways, more different than alike. But we all have a passion to shed light on the truth. Each of us, to the best of our ability, is doing what we can to enlighten those in our sphere of influence and bring a healing to this planet."

There was a long silence before his voice spoke again.

"There must be harmony between who a person is and what a person does. Passion for work can exist only when that work is a true reflection of one's beliefs and values."

"I used to believe that I could change the world with a song. I had passion then."

"And now?"

"Gone. I've lost it."

"No, not lost. Misplaced. It's time for you to channel it in a new direction."

"But, how? I've done one thing my whole life, and I don't know if I can do anything else."

"Tell me why you went into music."

"I wanted to communicate with the world, bring something beautiful to it."

"You loved making music, didn't you?"

"More than anything."

There was another long pause.

"Do you remember what I called the energy that flows through the biofield?"

"You called it love."

"Well, it's time for you to fall in love again, to fall in love with the highest vision of your self that you can imagine."

I took a deep breath and emptied my mind, but nothing came.

"The message you are waiting for isn't received with your mind. You receive it with your heart. Open your heart, son. Let the love flow through you."

I began to shut down, unwilling to go to that vulnerable place.

"I've got you, boy. You're safe with me. It's time to trust again, time to let go."

I took another deep breath, directing the flow of air into the middle of my chest. A flood of old feelings welled up in me. And when I exhaled, pain and fear I'd carried my whole life flowed out in a wash of tears.

When I finally sat upright again, peaceful warmth radiated from my chest into my head. And suddenly I could see a future me, telling stories, weaving in all I'd learned from Nate. At first I thought I was speaking to one person, but when I looked up, there were many. An unbroken chain.

"I can see it," I said out loud.

There was no response.

"*Thank you, Nate,*" my inner voice said.

"*It has been a pleasure.*"

"*When are you coming home?*"

"*Soon—there's still plenty of work for us to do.*"

"*Nate, are you really*"—I had to search for the right words—"*here with me?*"

"*Yes, son,*" he said, his voice fading, as the wind caught the edge of my smooth twig and sent it rolling down the rock.

"*But, how...?*"

"*That, my boy, is a lesson for another time.*"

AFTERWORD

Twenty years have passed since my first, eye-opening lesson with Nate. In that time, I've had the privilege of guiding thousands of individuals on their quests for better health. Each has had a unique set of challenges, but all possessed one thing in common: a willingness to change.

We humans resist change. For many, it is challenging and frightening—the doorway to the great unknown. But change is absolutely necessary for tomorrow to be better than today.

You and I are not so different. We are both products of a culture that promotes health care over self-care, convenience over quality, distraction over introspection. Maybe you too are one of the "walking wounded," not yet suffering from any particular disease but certainly not feeling your best.

Our time has been labeled the "Information Age," and we are presumably among the most well-informed humans ever to walk the Earth. But under Nate's tutelage, I came to realize how very little we actually know about the proper care and feeding of our bodies.

The man-made world bears little resemblance to the one nature designed. Those of us living in the artificial environments of suburbs and cities are like animals in a zoo, out of touch with the instincts necessary to thrive.

As a result, we have lost our sense of balance and have stumbled outside the boundaries nature established for us. The diseases that plague modern man are nothing more than reflections of this. For beyond those boundaries, monsters lurk: cardio-vascular disease, cancer, diabetes, Alzheimer's, and a host of other unnatural, chronic, degenerative conditions for which there are no medical cures.

Like it or not, the human body belongs to the natural world and is subject to natural law. When we break that law, and most of us do so daily, our bodies suffer the consequences.

The purpose of this story is to demonstrate that change is not only possible, but necessary if we wish to improve our health and the health of our planet. The concepts revealed here are not new. In some deep place, you already knew them.

The principles are simple and straightforward. Truth often is.

Nate opened my eyes to a series of fundamental truths about the way the world—the real world—works. But before I could see them, I had to let go of old beliefs and commonly held misperceptions—products of what Nate would call "mass consciousness." To see them, you'll need to let go too.

I assure you, the effort is worth making.

For information about Sam Rose's

Nutritional Consultations

Seminars

Recordings

(310) 473-8835

www.thewayback.com

www.rosenutrition.com

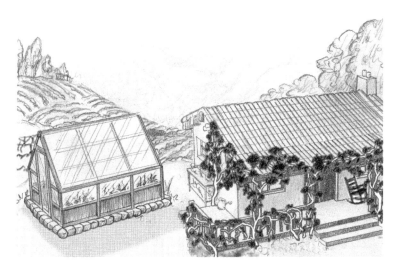

Made in the USA
Las Vegas, NV
12 September 2022

55180111R00184